Headache

in Primary Care

Headache

in Primary Care

Stephen D. Silberstein MD FACP
Thomas Jefferson University Headache Center,
Philadelphia, USA

Richard B. Lipton MD
Department of Neurology, Albert Einstein College of Medicine,
New York, USA

Peter J. Goadsby MD PhD DSc FRACP FRCP
Institute of Neurology, The National Hospital for
Neurology and Neurosurgery, London, UK

and

Robert T. Smith MD FAAFP FRCGP
Department of Family Medicine, University of Cincinnati,
Ohio, USA

I S I S
MEDICAL
MEDIA

Cover illustration by Jane McCormick

First published 1999

British Library Cataloguing in Publication Data.
A catalogue record for this title is available from the British Library

ISBN 1 901865 66 5

Silberstein, S D (Stephen)
Headache in Primary Care
S D Silberstein, R B Lipton, P J Goadsby (eds)

Always refer to the manufacturer's Prescribing Information before prescribing drugs cited in this book.

Design and Illustration by
InPerspective, London, UK

Isis Medical Media staff
Commissioning Editor: Jonathan Gregory
Editorial Controller: Fiona Cornell
Production Assistant: Sarah Sodhi

Printed and bound by
Sun Fung Offset Binding Co. Ltd.
Printed in China

Distributed in the USA by
Books International Inc., PO Box 605,
Herndon, VA 20172, USA

Distributed in the rest of the world by
Plymbridge Distributors Ltd., Estover Road,
Plymouth, PL6 7PY, UK

Contents

Preface

Headache is a universal human experience. For some people, headache is an occasional, episodic nuisance symptom. For others, it may be a manifestation of a disabling chronic disease or the first manifestation of a life-threatening condition. The cause, frequency, severity, and life consequences of headache vary widely. In this book, we have tried to systematically review current concepts of headache and its treatment, emphasizing the patient and the physician in the primary care setting.

Headache is a leading reason for consultation in primary care. Although the headache patients' treatment needs differ, the first step to successful management is a confident, credible, specific diagnosis. Patients often fear that their headaches are symptomatic of a serious underlying disorder such as a brain tumor. The primary care physician must distinguish primary headache disorders, such as migraine or tension-type headache, from secondary headaches, such as those resulting from brain mass lesion, infection, or metabolic derangement. For this reason, we discuss diagnosis and the utility of diagnostic tests in detail, devoting individual chapters to primary and secondary headaches.

The mysteries of headache are slowly being unlocked, due in large part to technology that allows researchers to study cerebral blood flow, the neuronal processes, electrophysiological and biochemical brain function, and genetic influences. The cause of a rare form of migraine, familial hemiplegic migraine, has been localized to chromosome 19, and the gene has been cloned. Functional neuroimaging has allowed us to see the brain centers intimately involved in the migraine attack. Epidemiologic studies that describe the prevalence of headache disorders and its coexistence with other conditions also contribute to our therapeutic approaches. We are gaining insight into the mechanisms of pain for the primary headache disorders. For the secondary headache disorders, we have long known that pain can be caused by inflammation, traction, or nerve root irritation from intracranial processes. This book describes the current state of headache science and reviews the mechanisms of primary and secondary headache disorders.

Our goal is to provide the primary care provider with a rigorous, accurate, practical approach to headache. We have devoted our careers to studying headache and improving patient care. With this book, we hope to provide the information and tools that our primary care colleagues need to better understand the headache patient and to make effective therapeutic decisions.

Stephen D. Silberstein
Richard B. Lipton
Peter J. Goadsby
Robert T. Smith

Acknowledgements

The authors would like to thank Joanne F. Okagaki for writing, editing, and project management and Lynne Kaiser for her editorial support.

1 The importance of headache in primary care practice

In primary care, patients with headache are seen more frequently than are patients with bronchitis, emphysema, or peptic ulcer disease. Individuals with migraine who seek medical help are more likely to consult a family physician or general practitioner than any other type of physician. Remarkable recent advances in the headache field have greatly increased the role that the primary care physician can play in raising the standards of headache care, and the aim of this book is to assist in achieving this goal.

Headache diagnosis

Scattered among the myriad clinical problems seen in primary care practice are many undifferentiated headaches. Accurate diagnosis, which is the cornerstone of good medical care, can be a challenge for the practitioner working under the time constraints and other pressures of a busy office practice. The diagnostic system based on headache classification devised by the International Headache Society (IHS) contributes greatly to more accurate diagnosis and clarifies previously vague headache diagnostic criteria.

The IHS system, first published in 1988, is widely accepted as the standard by headache experts. It divides headaches into 12 groups and further subdivides these groups in hierarchical fashion into subgroups that identify 129 different headaches, headache disorders, cranial neuralgias, and facial pains, any of which may present in primary care practice. However, the IHS classification system includes many rare and obscure conditions to meet the needs of specialists and researchers and does not highlight the more common headaches usually seen in primary care, and so it is cumbersome for use in routine practice. Chapter 2 in this book presents a more useful approach to classification without sacrificing any benefits of the IHS system. All headaches are assembled into two major areas:

- primary headaches, in which headache syndromes are the disease (IHS groups 1–4); and
- secondary headaches, in which other processes cause the headaches (IHS groups 5–12).

Primary headache disorders

Primary headaches consist of migraine, tension-type headache, cluster headache, and a miscellaneous group of headaches that occur less frequently. These recurrent and benign headaches constitute the major realm of the primary care physician's headache responsibilities (*see* Chapters 6–9), but the significance of secondary headaches in the primary care arena is certainly not less important. Although secondary headaches occur less frequently, a vital part of the primary care diagnostic process is knowing when to suspect headache caused by underlying pathology or associated systemic illness and when to refer the patient (*see* Chapter 10–15).

Primary care physicians have limited time available for each patient visit. Time may be further eroded as the physician deals with the headache patient's other concurrent health problems, which primary care studies show frequently include hypertension, depression, or diabetes. Primary care physicians are usually very familiar with their patients' health problems – a typical primary care patient has attended the same practice for five to six years, and visited the same physicians four or five times a year. Continuity of care, providing repeated opportunities for patient evaluation, reviewing progress, and maintaining the doctor–patient relationship are basic features of primary care practice, which makes it ideally suited for the care of headache patients. For physicians who are well prepared to deal with headache problems, repeated interactions with patients help to compensate for any brevity of individual visits.

Secondary headache disorders

Secondary headaches have many causes and, although rarely seen in primary care practice, it is possible that a patient may present with such a headache. Being aware of this possibility can help to avert serious diagnostic errors. However, to identify the underlying causes of these headaches can pose diagnostic difficulties beyond the scope of primary care practice (*see* Chapter 4).

Headache referral

Headache specialization is a relatively new field. The number of headache clinics and centres is growing, as are headache educational and research organizations that encourage the participation of primary care physicians. Although primary care physicians can now provide more effective care for headache patients than at any time in the past, knowing when to consult or refer to a neurologist or a headache specialist is essential for good primary care practice.

Headache patients in primary care are twice as likely to be referred than are non-headache patients. The most common cause for referral is chronic daily headache (CDH) that usually evolves from migraine or tension-type headache. Excessive use of analgesics, ergotamine preparations, or triptan is the main cause or significant aggravating factor of this problem. Much can be done at the primary care level to prevent CDH, and thereby reduce the need for specialty referral and hospital inpatient care (*see* Chapter 8). Careful maintenance of prescription records, monitoring drug use, and discouraging out-of-hours telephone calls for analgesic refills are measures that would greatly help reduce the problem. Patients with analgesic rebound headache (*see* Chapter 6) who overuse medication, go to great lengths, using ingenious and sometimes illegal methods, to obtain extra medication. Referral to a headache clinic with multispecialty services is necessary in such cases.

Headache danger signals

Headache severity is a poor indication of severe underlying pathology, as secondary headache may range in severity from mild discomfort to overwhelming agony. Primary care physicians should be familiar with the danger signals that suggest secondary headache (*see* Chapter 4). The physician should be alert to possible dangers when the patient reports 'the worst headache I've ever had', has changes in headache pattern, or presents with sustained headaches of severe and abrupt onset. Headache accompanied by neurological signs and symptoms other than aura and chronic headache in patients who have systemic illness or diseases known to spread intracranially should always raise suspicions. All headache patients should be examined neurologically when seen initially and again as necessary during repeat visits. Relying on headache history alone may have serious consequences, because a secondary headache may superimpose itself on a correctly diagnosed previous benign headache. Time constraints are not a valid reason for omitting a neurological examination and possibly missing a serious cause of headache.

Neurological screening in primary care

A neurological examination, which is an important part of headache assessment, begins as the patient enters the consulting room and greets the physician. Normal gait, facial expression, speech, cognition, appropriate behaviour, personal hygiene, and appropriate dress are all valuable indicators of likely normal cerebral functioning and the absence of major cerebral pathology.

Physicians skilled in performing a routine physical examination can quickly proceed with further neurological screening. The examination should:

- check eye movements, pupillary size, and fundi;
- check for papilloedema and retinal changes;
- test accommodation and light reflexes;
- do simple finger testing for loss in visual fields;
- examine upper and lower limbs for tremor, normal power, and tendon reflexes; and

• check for normal down-going plantar responses, normal finger-to-nose testing (to test cerebellar function), and stability when standing with eyes closed (Romberg's test).

Mental status is ascertained when taking the history. The addition of simple tests of recall completes the examination (*see* Chapter 4).

Imaging and headache diagnosis

Although computed tomography (CT) scanning and magnetic resonance imaging (MRI) are frequently carried out as part of the headache diagnosis process, they should not replace careful history taking and physical examination. Fear of missing underlying disease, demands from patients, and malpractice anxiety result in their overuse, even though the yield of these costly investigations is very low. If the primary care physician is convinced that after a thorough history and examination these tests are necessary, a specialist consultation is probably warranted. If the clinical need for such testing is urgent and consultation is not readily available, knowledge of the appropriate testing and immediate treatment steps to take is important (*see* Chapter 4).

Brain tumour and ruptured cerebral aneurysm are rare but commonly feared possibilities when a patient presents with sudden, unusually severe headache. Many brain tumours do not cause headache or may produce headaches that are indistinguishable from mild tension-type headache. In contrast, a subarachnoid haemorrhage caused by ruptured aneurysm is usually immediately apparent as a catastrophic intracranial event. Sentinel or premonitory headaches are usually caused by leakage from the aneurysm prior to major rupture. The hallmark is headache of very sudden onset, with or without associated neurological symptoms, that waxes and wanes over days or even weeks. If suspected, this requires urgent specialty referral.

Headache treatment

Most headache sufferers do not consult a physician even when suffering from severe treatable headaches. Thus, the primary care physician has a major role to play in increasing public awareness of the availability of effective headache treatments. Headache patients first consult a doctor for a variety of reasons:

• to improve their self-treatment methods;
• worsening symptoms or a growing fear of underlying disease;
• pressure from family members and friends; or
• information from the media that promotes headache care and new drugs.

Patient expectations of a cure for their headache need to be replaced by an understanding that the treatment goal is headache control. Optimal care begins with an empathetic physician who has effective communication skills, takes a careful history, performs a physical examination, explains the nature of the problem, and affirms that it is not 'all in your head'. The importance of patient education needs to be stressed, as does the active partnership role the patients must play in their treatment.

A wide range of non-prescription and prescription drugs is available to treat headache. With the introduction of the triptans, many new treatment options are now available (*see* tables in Chapter 6). Patient compliance and strict adherence to the recommended drug regimen is essential for good management, as are clear instructions about practice arrangements, prescription refills, future visits, and out-of-hours calls.

Increasing knowledge of the underlying mechanisms is adding scientific principles to the art of headache care (*see* Chapter 5), and headache has become a fast-growing branch of the neurosciences. Primary care physicians require more information about these developments and need to become more aware of how these developments may benefit their patients, particularly in terms of providing a more coherent explanation of their symptoms and treatment.

Traditionally, medical students and residents are given little training in headache. Primary care physicians first entering practice are often poorly prepared to deal adequately with the complex headache problems they confront in practice. Headache education for the general practitioner is haphazard, mainly accomplished through specialty consultations and periodic attendance at continuing education programs. General economic constraints in the health field and the pressures of managed care assure that the main clinical burden of dealing with headaches will continue to be carried, not by neurologists or headache specialists, but by primary care physicians, and this pattern is unlikely to change in the near future. Thus, the initiative to improve headache care is, and will remain, in the hands of the practitioner. This book is designed to help the physician who is willing to take the initiative to meet the headache challenge in primary care.

Further reading

Smith R. American Academy of Family Physicians. *Headache.* Monograph 203. Home Study Self-Assessment. American Academy of Family Physicians, 1996.

Headache Classification Committee of the International Headache Society. Classification and diagnostic criteria for headache disorders, cranial neuralgias and facial pain. *Cephalalgia* 1988; 8 (Suppl. 7): 1–96.

Lipton RB, Stewart WF, Simon D. Medical consultation for migraine: results from the American Migraine Study. *Headache* 1998; 38(2): 87–96.

Mathew NT. Drug-induced headache. *Neurol Clin* 1990; 8: 903–12.

Mitchell CS, Osborne RE, Grosskrentz SR. Computed tomography in the headache patient: is routine evaluation really necessary? *Headache* 1993; 33: 82–6.

Stange CK, Zyzanski SJ, Jaen CR, Callahan EJ. Illuminating the 'Black Box' – a description of patient visits to family physicians. *J Fam Pract* 1998; 46(5): 377–69.

Pathophysiology and epidemiology of headache

2 Classification and diagnosis of headache

Introduction

Headache, like back pain or abdominal pain, is a symptom that can have many causes. Headache may occur in relative isolation, as part of an acute symptom complex (e.g. migraine or cluster headaches), or as part of an evolving disorder (e.g. brain tumour or Lyme disease). Since a range of disorders produce headache, a systematic approach to headache classification and diagnosis is an essential prelude to its management and treatment. In this chapter, contemporary approaches to headache classification and diagnosis are reviewed.

The 1988 International Headache Society (IHS) classification of headache (Table 2.1) established consistent terminology and diagnostic criteria for headache. This classification system is almost universally accepted and has become the basis for headache classification in the International Classification of Diseases (ICD-10b). The IHS system first distinguishes primary and secondary headache disorders. Secondary headaches are symptomatic of an underlying cause, like brain tumour, temporal arteritis, or infection. In primary headaches, there is no underlying illness. The IHS criteria further divide primary headache disorders into four major categories (Table 2.1-A) and into nine major categories of secondary headache disorders (Table 2.1-B). A patient may have more than one headache disorder, so these criteria are intended to describe headache types, not patients. In the IHS system, primary headaches are classified based on symptom profiles, since the underlying causes for primary headache are not precisely known. However, secondary headaches are classified by underlying causes.

● **Table 2.1** The IHS classification system

A Primary headache disorders	B Secondary headache disorders
1 Migraine	**5** Headache associated with head trauma
1.1 Migraine without aura	5.1 Acute post-traumatic headache
1.2 Migraine with aura	5.2 Chronic post-traumatic headache
1.3 Ophthalmoplegic	**6** Headache associated with vascular disorders
2 Tension-type headache	**7** Headache associated with non-vascular intracranial disorder
2.1 Episodic tension-type headache	7.1 High cerebrospinal fluid pressure
2.2 Chronic tension-type headache	7.2 Low cerebrospinal fluid pressure
3 Cluster headache and chronic paroxysmal hemicrania	7.3 Intracranial infection
3.1 Cluster headache	7.4 Intracranial sarcoidosis and other non-infectious inflammatory diseases
3.1.1 Episodic cluster headache	7.5 Headache related to intrathecal injections
3.1.2 Chronic cluster headache	7.6 Intracranial neoplasm
3.2 Chronic paroxysmal hemicrania	**8** Headache associated with substances or their withdrawal
4 Miscellaneous headaches unassociated with structural lesion	**9** Headache associated with non-cephalic infection
4.1 Idiopathic stabbing headache	9.1 Viral infection
4.2 External compression headache	9.2 Bacterial infection
4.3 Cold stimulus headache	9.3 Headache related to other infection
4.4 Benign cough headache	**10** Headache associated with metabolic disorder
4.5 Benign exertional headache	**11** Headache or facial pain associated with disorder of the cranium, neck, eyes, ears, nose, sinuses, teeth, mouth or other facial or cranial structures
4.6 Headache associated with sexual activity	**12** Cranial neuralgias, nerve trunk pain and deafferentation pain
Headache Classification Committee of the IHS, 1988	**13** Headache not classifiable

Clinical approach: an overview

In evaluating a headache patient, the first task is to identify or exclude secondary headache. This decision is based on the patient's history and the general medical and neurological examinations (Figure 2.1). Important aspects of the headache history are summarized in Table 2.2. If suspicious features are present, diagnostic testing may be necessary (Table 2.3). Once secondary headaches have been excluded, the task is to diagnose one or more specific primary headache disorders. In the initial evaluation, the physician should look for 'headache alarms' that could signal a secondary headache disorder. Table 2.3 summarizes these alarms, suggests

● **Table 2.2** *Headache history*

Attack onset

Pain location

Attack duration

Attack frequency and timing

Pain severity

Pain quality

Associated features

Aggravating or precipitating factors

Ameliorating factors

Social history

Family history

Past headache history

Headache impact

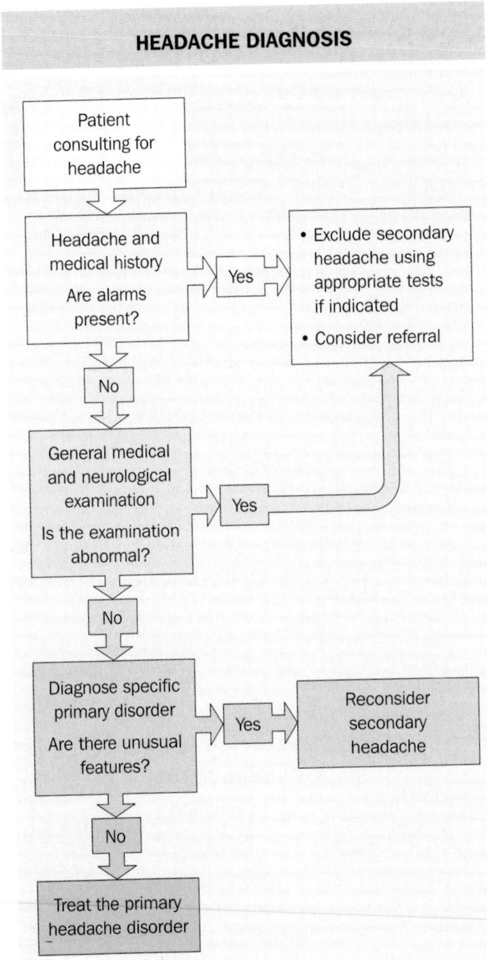

HEADACHE DIAGNOSIS

● **Figure 2.1** *Core algorithm for headache diagnosis.*

● **Table 2.3** *Diagnostic alarms in the evaluation of headache disorders*

Headache alarm	Differential diagnosis	Possible work-up
Headache begins after the age of 50 years	Temporal arteritis, mass lesion	Erythrocyte sedimentation rate, neuroimaging
Sudden-onset headache	Subarachnoid haemorrhage, pituitary apoplexy, bleed into a mass or arteriovenous malformation, mass lesion (especially posterior fossa)	Neuroimaging, lumbar puncture
Accelerating pattern of headaches	Mass lesion, subdural haematoma, medication overuse	Neuroimaging, drug screen
New-onset headache in a patient with cancer or human immunodeficiency virus	Meningitis (chronic or carcinomatous), brain abscess (including toxoplasmosis), metastasis	Neuroimaging, lumbar puncture
Headache with systemic illness (fever, stiff neck, rash)	Meningitis, encephalitis, Lyme disease, systemic infection, collagen vascular disease	Neuroimaging, lumbar puncture, blood tests
Focal neurological symptoms or signs of disease (other than typical aura)	Mass lesion, arteriovenous malformation, stroke, collagen vascular disease (including antiphospholipid antibodies)	Neuroimaging, collagen vascular evaluation
Papilloedema	Mass lesion, pseudotumour, meningitis	Neuroimaging, lumbar puncture

a possible differential diagnosis for each, and lists a possible work-up. Recent studies demonstrate that computed tomography (CT) and magnetic resonance imaging (MRI) of the head yield extremely few abnormal findings among headache patients if 'alarms' based on the history and physical examinations are lacking. In Chapter 4, diagnostic testing is reviewed in detail. If patients do not fit neatly into the IHS diagnostic categories or if response to treatment is atypical, the physician should re-evaluate the patient for secondary headache.

Headache history

Overview

Most headache patients have normal medical and neurological examinations. Therefore, a careful history becomes the most important tool for accurate diagnosis. The history should provide a comprehensive view of the patient's headaches as well as any associated conditions or problems that could influence diagnosis and treatment (Table 2.2). Not only is the history essential for diagnosis, but the time spent helps to establish rapport with the patient, who is often fearful that the headaches have a life-threatening cause. In primary care, many headache patients have a long-standing relationship with the physician, which facilitates a rapid, thorough, and mutually satisfactory interaction. Time spent on the history and physical examination has a therapeutic as well as a diagnostic function.

The clinician should first ask the patient to give an unstructured account of the problem ('Tell me about your headaches'), then systematically explore the various headache features and patterns. Since many patients have more than one type of headache and the pattern may change over time, the patient should usually begin by describing the headache of most concern or the one that motivated the consultation. A questionnaire that patients complete prior to the consultation helps them to focus on symptoms and improves the reliability and efficiency of the history.

Once secondary headaches have been excluded, we recommend the use of a brief questionnaire to ascertain some key elements of the headache history. One such questionnaire, The Headache Evaluation Questionnaire, is shown in Figure 2.2.

The following sections of this chapter describe headache features that help with the differential diagnosis – onset, location, duration, frequency and/or timing, severity, quality, and associated features (Table 2.4).

Headache onset

The age and context of headache onset provides important clues for diagnosis. Possible patterns include:

- onset in childhood or early adult life – primary headaches usually begin at this time;
- onset after 55 years of age – could indicate more serious disorders (mass lesions or giant cell arteritis);
- onset after head injury – suggest post-concussive headache disorder or intracranial pathology (however, migraine and cluster headache may also be triggered by head trauma);
- onset during peripartum period – may result from cortical vein or sagittal sinus thromboses;
- onset with fever – suggests infectious aetiology; or
- onset with exertion – suggests subarachnoid haemorrhage or other serious causes as well as benign exertional headache.

Location and duration of pain

The location of pain at onset and the way it spreads assists diagnosis because many headaches follow typical pain patterns:

- Migraine – unilateral, hemicranial pain that may change sides from attack to attack, but pain often has a predilection for one side. Migraine may be bilateral in 20–30% of adults and in a higher proportion of children.
- Cluster headache – almost always unilateral pain that occurs in or around one eye, the temple, or adjacent areas. 15–20% of cluster patients report that pain changes side from one cluster period to the next. Rarely, cluster changes sides within a cluster period.

HEADACHE EVALUATION QUESTIONNAIRE

Instructions: This questionnaire helps evaluate the headaches you have had in the *past 3 months*. Please answer every question as best you can in the space provided.

Name   Age   Sex: Female   Male   Today's date:

1 What would you like us to know about your headaches? (Tick all the answers that apply.)

a   I want you to know about my headaches, but I don't need help right now.

b   I would like help about my headaches this visit.

c   My headaches are the main reason for this visit.

d   I am very worried about my overall health because of my headaches.

e   Other   Please describe:

2 Has your doctor ever told you what kind of headache you have?

If Yes, what did your doctor call your headache?   Cluster   Migraine   Tension   Other:

If No, what kind of headache do you think you have?   Cluster   Migraine   Tension   Other:

3 During the *past 3 months*, how many days did you have headache?   Days

4 During the *past 3 months*, how many days did your headaches limit you from working, studying, or carrying on your usual activities?   Days

5 During the *past 3 months*, how many days have you taken the following drugs? (Please write '0' for none.)

Over-the-counter (OTC) drugs		Drugs prescribed by a doctor			
Advil®	Days	Amerge®	Days	Vicodin®	Days
Aleve®	Days	Cafergot®	Days	Wigraine®	Days
Aspirin	Days	Fioricet®	Days	Zomig®	Days
Excedrin®	Days	Fiorinal®	Days	Other prescription drugs	Days
Motrin®	Days	Imitrex®	Days	Specify	
Nuprin®	Days	Maxalt®	Days		
Tylenol®	Days	Midrin®	Days		
Other OTC drugs	Days	Tylenol® with codeine	Days		
Specify					

6 During the *past 3 months*, has the pain, number of your headaches, or concern about your headaches changed?   Yes   No

If Yes, tick the answers that apply to the *past 3 months*, as compared with other times before:

a The pain of my headaches has: Decreased   Remained the same   Increased   Significantly increased

b The number of my headaches has: Decreased   Remained the same   Increased   Significantly increased

c The worry, trouble, or anxiety caused by my headaches has: Decreased   Remained the same   Increased   Significantly increased

7 For *each* of the following statements, tick how often each type of pain was associated with your headaches during the *past 3 months*.

	Never	Rarely	Less than half the time	More than half the time
a The pain was worse on just one side				
b The pain was pounding, pulsing, or throbbing				
c The pain was moderate or severe				
d The pain was made worse by routine activities such as walking or climbing stairs				

8 For *each* of the following statements, tick how often you felt discomfort with your headaches during the *past 3 months*.

	Never	Rarely	Less than half the time	More than half the time
a You felt nauseated or sick to your stomach				
b You saw spots, stars, zig-zags, lines, or grey areas continuously for several minutes or more during or before your headaches				
c Light bothered you (a lot more than when you don't have headaches)				
d Sound bothered you (a lot more than when you don't have headaches)				

●**Figure 2.2** *Headache evaluation questionnaire.*

● **Table 2.4** *Differential diagnosis of selected headache disorders*

Headache type	Age of onset (years)	Location	Duration	Frequency/ timing	Severity	Quality	Associated Features
Migraine	10–40	Hemicranial	4–72 hours	Variable	Moderate– severe	Throbbing > steady ache	Nausea, vomiting, photo/phono/ osmophobia, scotomata, neurological deficits
Tension type	20–50	Bilateral	30 min to 7 days +	Variable	Dull ache may wax/ wane	Vice-like, band-like pressure	Generally none
Cluster	15–40	Unilateral peri/retro- orbital	15–180 min	1–8 times per day, nocturnal attacks	Excruciating	Boring piercing	Ipsilateral conjunctival injection, lacrimation, nasal congestion, rhinorrhoea, miosis, facial sweating
Mass lesion	Any	Any	Variable	Intermittent, nocturnal, upon arising	Moderate	Dull steady/ throbbing	Vomiting, nuchal rigidity, neurological deficits
Subarachnoid haemorrhage	Adult	Global, often occipitonuchal	Variable	Not applicable	Excruciating	Explosive	Nausea, vomiting, nuchal rigidity, loss of consciousness, neurological deficits
Trigeminal neuralgia	50–70	2nd–3rd > 1st division's trigeminal nerve	Seconds, occur in volleys	Paroxysmal	Excruciating	Electric shock-like	Facial trigger points, spasm of muscles ipsilaterally (Tic)
Giant cell arteritis	>55	Temporal, any region	Intermittent, then contin- uous	Constant, ? worse at night	Variable	Variable	Tender scalp arteries, polymyalgia rheumatica, jaw claudication

- Tension-type headache – bilateral pain in 60% of cases, usually distribution is bifrontal, bioccipital, or as a hatband.
- Headache from organic disease – may have localized pain. (For example, periorbital pain may indicate ocular pathology; face pain may indicate trigeminal neuralgia.) More than 50% of patients with brain tumour have headache, and 80% of those have pain on the side of the tumour.

Pain duration also provides clues for diagnosis (Table 2.4):

- 4–72 hours – typical for migraine (migraines that last >72 hours are termed 'status migrainosus');
- 15–180 minutes – typical for cluster headaches (range is 10 minutes to several hours);
- 5–20 minutes – typical for paroxysmal hemicrania (range is 1 minute to 120 minutes);
- 30 minutes to 7 days – typical for episodic tension-type headache;
- Headaches of organic origin do not have a characteristic duration.

Change in duration (for example, attacks last longer) suggests the need for diagnostic evaluation.

Frequency and timing of attacks
The frequency and timing of headaches help to determine both diagnosis and treatment. The physician should elicit the following information about temporal patterns from the patient:

- how often attacks occur;
- the longest headache-free period in the past 6 months;

- whether attacks are associated with menstrual cycle; and
- whether attacks are associated with specific temporal patterns – weekends, holidays, relaxing after stress.

The following list describes temporal patterns that may be seen with various types of headache:

- migraine attacks – may occur at random, with menstrual cycle, or with specific temporal patterns (weekends, holidays, relaxing after stress);
- episodic cluster headaches – typically occur in a regular pattern, with attacks recurring at similar times of the day or night, often waking the patient during rapid eye-movement (REM) sleep;
- episodic tension-type headaches – recur less than 15 times a month (those that occur more than 15 times a month are classified as chronic tension-type headache).

Headache patterns may suggest useful preventive strategies:

- menstrual migraines may respond to perimenstrual use of non-steroidal anti-inflammatory drugs (NSAIDs);
- nocturnal cluster attacks may be prevented by the administration of ergotamine at bedtime; and
- organic headaches may be episodic or daily and continuous – they do not occur with any set pattern and may mimic the known primary headaches.

Pain severity and quality

Pain severity and rapidity of onset and resolution are important clues for diagnosis. The physician can use a pain scale of 1 to 10 (1 is minimal discomfort, 10 the most excruciating pain the patient can imagine) that allows the patient to describe pain intensity within an individual attack and across attacks. This scale may not be fully comparable across patients, but it helps record an individual's progress. Among the primary headaches, pain is severe for migraine (median

pain is 8 out of 10), but less severe for tension-type headache (median pain is 3–4 out of 10).

Headaches of very sudden onset are worrisome. For example, the headache of subarachnoid haemorrhage classically has a sudden, explosive onset (Table 2.3).

The quality of pain provides diagnostic clues (Table 2.4):

- migraine – throbbing or pulsatile, often begins as a dull, steady ache that slowly evolves (may not throb until pain becomes moderate to severe);
- cluster – deep, boring, or piercing, often likened to a red-hot poker thrust into the eye;
- tension-type – dull, band-like, vice-like;
- brain tumour headache – like tension-type (dull, band-like, vice-like); and
- ruptured aneurysm or arteriovenous malformation (AVM) headache – most often a continuous, intense, aching or throbbing pain.

Associated features

Associated symptoms or features may occur prior to, during, or following the headache. The details of associated symptoms are discussed in subsequent chapters on each type of headache. Taking care not to elicit false-positive responses, the physician should ask the patient whether he or she experiences any symptoms associated with the headache before, during, or after it occurs (the range of symptoms is listed in Table 2.4). The physician should distinguish between symptoms associated with the headache and those chronically present in that patient. For example, photophobia refers to an unusual or heightened sensitivity to light, and if the patient's photophobia is not specifically associated with headache, it should not be counted as an associated symptom.

Neurological deficits may accompany headaches that are caused by organic disease, depending on the location of the lesion. For example, intracranial mass lesions are associated with nausea and vomiting or, in half the cases, vomiting without nausea (projectile). Giant cell arteritis may be associated with localized scalp tenderness, malaise, arthralgias or myalgias, low-grade fevers, depression, or other constitutional symptoms.

Aggravating or precipitating factors (triggers)

Identifying factors or triggers that precipitate or aggravate headache attacks is useful in establishing a diagnosis, implementing a treatment programme, and avoiding attacks. Common triggers are:

- Migraine – menstruation, stress, relaxation after stress, fatigue, too much or too little sleep, skipping a meal, weather changes, high humidity, high altitude, exposure to glare or flickering lights, loud noises, perfumes or chemical fumes, postural changes, physical activity, or coughing. In addition, food triggers occur in 10% of migraineurs. These may include chocolate, cheese, alcoholic beverages (especially red wine), citrus fruits, and foods containing monosodium glutamate, nitrates, and aspartate. Cocaine use and withdrawal may also trigger a migraine-like headache.
- Cluster – ingesting alcohol during a cluster period, usually within 30 minutes after ingestion (during the remission phase of cluster, alcohol does not precipitate an attack). Lying down aggravates cluster.
- Tension-type – end of the day (aggravated by daily stress).
- Headache from trigeminal neuralgia – stimulation of trigger points of the face and mouth, such as eating, speaking, exposure to cold air, brushing the teeth, or stroking, shaving, or washing the face may provoke an attack.
- Headache from brain tumour – intensified by exertion, postural changes, bending over, or coughing.
- Aneurysmal rupture – may be precipitated by exertion associated with increased blood pressure, such as with sexual activity.

Ameliorating factors

Identifying the factors, both pharmacological and non-pharmacological, that ameliorate

headache pain and associated symptoms provides useful diagnostic and therapeutic information. Examples are:

- Migraine – retiring to a dark, quiet room and lying motionless; sleep; pressure on the superficial temporal artery (but only when being pressed); hot or cold compresses; frequency and severity often decrease during the last two trimesters of pregnancy or with the onset of menopause (also with cluster).
- Cluster – sitting upright, rocking in a chair, pacing, engaging in vigorous movement.
- Tension-type – relaxing, resting, or sleeping.
- Pharmacological factors may include using a drug erroneously (subtherapeutic dose, overuse, or abuse).

Social history

Social factors may play a significant role in headache. The clinician can explore the following aspects of the patient's life to find sources of stress:

- Patient's marital and family status, education, occupation, outside interests, and friendships.
- Major life change – marriage, divorce, separation, new job, retirement, or death in the family.
- Work related-stress – conflict in the workplace, type of employment, exposure to drugs or toxins, exposure to nitroglycerin (for example, in munitions factories), carbon monoxide.
- Sleep habits – sleep apnoea, which is common in middle-aged obese men, may cause morning headache; depression may make falling or staying asleep difficult or may waken the patient in the early morning; anxiety may make falling asleep difficult.
- Other habits – use of alcohol, tobacco, caffeine, or illicit drugs; a history of unprotected sex should prompt a search for potential infection.

Family history

Some headache disorders are familial. Approximately 50–60% of migraineurs have a parent with the disorder, and up to 80% have at least one first-degree relative with migraine. Of patients with tension-type headaches, 40% have family members with similar headaches, but cluster headaches rarely occur within the same family. Thus, obtaining a family history is useful, and ideally one from each affected relative directly; however, the patient's description of the family member's headache, including any associated features, can also be helpful.

Familial headaches do not necessarily imply a genetic basis, although this seems to be the case in migraine sufferers. Shared environmental exposures may be the cause of headaches within some families. For example, a family subject to a leaky furnace may suffer headaches caused by carbon monoxide. However, the very common co-occurrence of headaches within families is sometimes simply the result of chance.

Past headache history

Taking a history of medications and dosages, as previously described, is useful because:

- treatment response may help support a diagnosis;
- treatment failure may result from inadequate dosing and timing strategies (for example, discontinuing a beta-blocker after only a 1-week trial); and
- treatment benefits and side effects from the past can guide future treatment plans.

Reviewing the current approach to headache treatment with the patient can reveal wilful or unwitting overuse of over-the-counter pain relievers. Excessive use of drugs that contain caffeine, narcotics, barbiturates, and ergots can produce medication withdrawal or rebound headaches. Correction of medication overuse is an essential step towards improving headache control. Occasionally, outpatient treatment fails and specialist referral for inpatient management is required. Increasing subtherapeutic regimens into the therapeutic range may result in better headache control.

Asking about other non-drug therapies, such as psychotherapy, biofeedback, acupuncture, chiropractic therapy, or treatment with herbs, vitamin, or homeopathic remedies can be helpful. Biofeedback is often a useful modality. Understanding the patient's use of complementary methods can help the doctor identify useful or dangerous methods and better understand the patient's values and treatment preferences.

Patients with long-standing headaches may have had many diagnostic tests and taken a variety of medications. A reasonable effort to verify prior test results, obtaining copies of reports, can help with diagnosis and treatment strategy.

Headache-related disability

Diagnosis alone does not provide enough information about the primary headache disorders to optimize therapy. In addition to diagnosis, clinicians should consider the impact of the headache disorder on the patient's life. Some patients seek help primarily out of concern that the headache is symptomatic of a serious underlying disease. For these patients, reassurance may be the most important intervention. Other patients have severe pain and disability that require a programme of care to improve their lives. It is, therefore, important to ask patients how headaches affect their lives and what they were hoping for in seeking care. We recommend assessing headache disability using the Migraine Disability Assessment (MIDAS) questionnaire (Figure 2.3). This questionnaire measures over the past 3 months the effect of headache on work or school, household work, and family, social, and leisure activities. A MIDAS score greater than 10 defines a more disabled group of headache sufferers. This group accounts for a substantial portion of all work loss and is an excellent group to target for aggressive diagnostic and therapeutic intervention.

Physical and neurological examinations

While most patients with a chief complaint of headache have an entirely normal examination, this portion of the consultation must not be overlooked because it will help guide diagnosis and treatment strategies.

A thorough examination includes:

- vital signs;
- examination of the heart and lungs;

MIGRAINE DISABILITY ASSESSMENT (MIDAS) QUESTIONNAIRE

Instructions: Please answer the following questions about ALL your headaches you have had over the *past 3 months*. Write your answer in the box next to each question. Write '0' if you did not do the activity in the *past 3 months*.

1 On how many days in the *past 3 months* did you miss work or school because of your headaches?   days

2 How many days in the *past 3 months* was your productivity at work or school reduced by half or more because of your headaches? (*Do not include days you counted in question 1 when you missed work or school.*)   days

3 On how many days in the *past 3 months* did you not do household work because of your headaches?   days

4 How many days in the *past 3 months* was your productivity in household work reduced by half or more because of your headaches? (*Do not include days you counted in question 3 when you missed work or school.*)   days

5 How many days in the *past 3 months* did you miss family, social, or leisure activities because of your headaches?   days

---

MIDAS score

A On how many days in the *past 3 months* did you have a headache? (*If a headache lasted more than 1 day, count each day.*)   days

B On a scale of 0–10 how painful were these headaches? (*Where 0 = no pain at all, and 10 = pain as bad as it can be.*)

© Innovative Medical Research

● **Figure 2.3** *Migraine disability assessment (MIDAS) questionnaire.*

- auscultation of the carotid and vertebral arteries, looking for bruits;
- palpation of head and neck, looking for trigger points, other tender areas, masses, bruises, or thickened blood vessels; and
- checking the temporomandibular joint for tenderness, decreased mobility, asymmetry, or 'clicking.'

A few key signs in the neurological examination bear emphasis:

- evidence of papilloedema – suggests increased intracranial pressure and warrants an imaging procedure to rule out a mass lesion (the key early features of papilloedema are loss of spontaneous venous pulsations and venous engorgement);
- nuchal rigidity because of meningeal irritation – seen with meningitis, intracerebral mass lesions, and intraparenchymal or subarachnoid haemorrhages, and prompts a rapid work-up;
- focal neurological deficits – may indicate structural brain disease and requires neuroimaging;

- thickened or nodular temporal artery, diminished or absent temporal artery pulsations, reddened, tender scalp nodules, or necrotic lesions of the scalp or tongue – indicate giant cell arteritis;
- Horner's syndrome (ptosis and miosis) – may be seen with cluster headaches, chronic paroxysmal hemicrania, as well as carotid and or intracranial lesions.

History after the initial visit

A diagnosis may not be established on the first visit, or perhaps an initial assessment may be incorrect. It is often useful to ask the patient to keep a headache diary to record the date, severity, duration, and associated features of each headache attack, as well as the medications used and the possible triggers. On subsequent visits, reviewing the diary may uncover previously unrecognized patterns that can provide clues in diagnosis and suggest treatment. Diaries also increase the efficiency of follow-up visits by providing accurate summaries, which can be grouped at a glance, as opposed to painstaking and less accurate histories.

Summary

- Besides defining headache types, the IHS classification system helps the physician to organize information about clinical features and laboratory tests, a process necessary for diagnosis and to plan treatment strategies.
- In evaluating a headache patient, the first task is to identify or exclude secondary headache, which is a decision based on a thorough physical examination and history.
- Most headache patients have a normal medical and neurological examination. Therefore, a comprehensive history becomes the most important tool for accurate diagnosis and effective treatment.
- Obtaining a complete and accurate history is an art that takes practice. Although time-consuming and often frustrating, time invested facilitates diagnosis and treatment and helps to allay fears.
- Age at onset, location of pain and its duration, frequency and/or timing, severity, quality, and associated features all provide clues that aid diagnosis and guide treatment.
- The patient's social and family history, triggers, and ameliorating factors help the physician to understand the nature of the headaches.
- When the primary care physician suspects a secondary cause of headache, detection and diagnosis may be a matter for the specialist consultant.

Further reading

Dalessio DJ, Silberstein SD. Diagnosis and classificaton of headache. In: *Wolff's Headache and Other Head Pain,* 6th edn. New York: Oxford University Press, 1993: 3–18.

Edmeads J. Emergency management of headache. *Headache* 1988; 28: 675–9.

Headache Classification Committee of the International Headache Society. Classification and diagnostic criteria for headache disorders, cranial neuralgia, and facial pain. *Cephalalgia* 1988; 8 (Suppl. 7): 1–96.

Prysé-Phillips WEM, Dodick DW, Edmeads JG *et al.* Guidelines for the diagnosis of migraine in clinical practice. *Can Med Assoc J* 1997; 156(9): 1273–87.

Quality Standards Subcommittee of the American Academy of Neurology. Practice parameter: the utility of neuroimaging in the evaluation of headache in patients with normal neurologic examinations (summary statement). *Neurology* 1994; 44: 1353–4.

Silberstein SD. Evaluation and emergency treatment of headache. *Headache* 1992; 32: 396–407.

3 Epidemiology and impact of headache disorders

Introduction

Epidemiology impacts the diagnosis and treatment of headache disorders by providing insights into their distribution in the population. Social, familial, and environmental risk factors that influence headache prevalence can provide clues to the cause of headache and assist in its classification. Conditions that are comorbid with specific headache disorders (i.e. occur at a higher frequency than would be expected) have been identified. The presence of a comorbid disorder profoundly influences headache diagnosis and treatment.

Epidemiological studies evaluate individuals in the population whether or not they are within the health system. This is important because each year only a small minority of headache sufferers ever see a doctor. In the United States, less than half of migraine sufferers sought medical care in 1998. Clinic-based studies, therefore, introduce a selection bias that limits the ability to generalize and may alter research results. In this chapter, studies of primary headache disorders carried out in the general population (population-based) are reviewed. Since case definition influences results, only studies that use the International Headache Society (IHS) criteria are discussed. Some key epidemiological terms are summarized in Table 3.1.

As there are no objective diagnostic tests for the diagnosis of primary headache disorders, diagnosis is based on symptom profile. The gold standard for headache diagnosis, the IHS criteria, is applied following a careful clinical evaluation. The IHS criteria define migraine and tension-type headache as distinct disorders; some headache specialists favour the 'spectrum' or 'continuum' concept. According to this view, migraine and tension-type headache exist as polar ends on a continuum of severity, and vary more in degree than in kind. We believe that migraine and tension-type headache are distinct disorders. However, when an individual with migraine also has tension-type headache, the two disorders in the same person may have related mechanisms. Differences in epidemiological profiles, patterns of family aggregation, symptom profile, and treatment

• **Table 3.1** *Definitions of epidemiological terms*

Reliability:	That independent diagnostic evaluations yield consistent diagnostic results.
Validity:	The assigned diagnosis is related to the underlying biology of the disorder.
Prevalence:	The proportion of a given population that has a disorder over a defined period of time.
Lifetime prevalence:	The proportion of individuals who have ever had the condition.
Period prevalence:	The proportion of individuals who have had at least one attack within a defined interval, usually within 1 year of the time of ascertainment.
Incidence:	The onset of new cases of a disease in a defined population over a given period of time

response suggest that migraine and pure tension-type headache are probably distinct.

Epidemiology of primary and secondary headache

In a landmark study, Rasmussen and coworkers examined the epidemiology of a broad range of headache disorders using the IHS criteria in a sample of nearly 1000 individuals in the greater Copenhagen area. The lifetime prevalence of various headache disorders is summarized in Table 3.2. The most common primary headache disorder was tension-type headache, followed by migraine. Of the secondary headache disorders, fasting (a headache precipitated by hunger) was the single most common, followed by headache caused by nose and/or sinus disease and headache from head trauma.

Epidemiology of migraine

Overall, the 1-year period prevalence of migraine in North America and Western Europe is about

● **Table 3.2** *Lifetime prevalence of headache*

Type	Prevalence (%)
Primary headache	
Tension-type headache	78
Migraine	16
Secondary headache	
Fasting	19
Nose and/or sinus disease	15
Head trauma	4
Non-vascular intracranial disease (including brain tumour)	0.5

After Rasmussen et al., 1991.

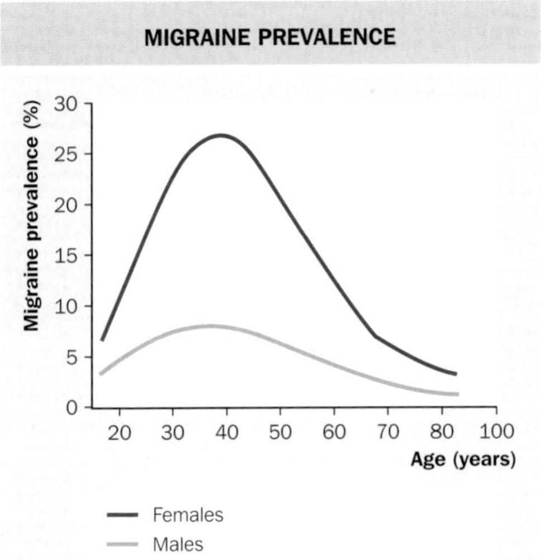

MIGRAINE PREVALENCE

● **Figure 3.1** *Age- and sex-specific prevalence of migraine. (From Stewart et al., 1992.)*

10%. Prevalence varies strikingly by age and gender. Before the age of 12 years, migraine is, if anything, more common in boys. At puberty, prevalence increases more rapidly in girls than boys, peaks at approximately 40 years of age, and declines thereafter (Figure 3.1). At all post-pubertal ages, overall migraine prevalence is about 18% in women and about 6% in men; thus, migraine is three times more common in females than in males.

Migraine prevalence is also influenced by race and geographical region. Prevalence is highest in North America and Western Europe, lower in Africa, and lower still in Asian countries. Patterns by race in the United States show that prevalence is highest in Caucasians, inter-mediate in African–Americans, and lowest in Asian–Americans. While these patterns require additional study, they are compatible with race-related genetic differences in migraine risk.

Comorbidity of migraine

Why study comorbidity?

Comorbidity refers to the more-than-coincidental association of two conditions in the same individual. Migraine is comorbid with stroke, epilepsy, depression, and anxiety disorders. Understanding comorbidity has important implications from a number of perspectives:

- Comorbidity has diagnostic implications when symptoms overlap. For example, both migraine and epilepsy can cause transient alterations of consciousness. The presence of migraine should increase the index of diagnostic suspicion for comorbid conditions, such as epilepsy, depression, and anxiety disorders. Similarly, in people with these conditions, it is important to look for migraine.
- Comorbid conditions have treatment implications because they can impose therapeutic limitations or create therapeutic opportunities. For example, migraine drugs that lower the seizure threshold must be used with caution in the patient with migraine and epilepsy; examples include the tricyclic antidepressants, selective serotonin re-uptake inhibitors, and neuroleptics. On the other hand, if migraine and depression occur together, an antidepressant can treat both conditions. Similarly, the anti-migraine/anti-epileptic agent, sodium valproate (divalproex sodium), can prevent attacks of both migraine and epilepsy.
- The study of comorbidity may provide clues to the fundamental mechanisms of migraine.

Migraine and stroke

A substantial body of literature links migraine and stroke, which appear together more often in migraine with aura and in stroke that involves the posterior circulation of the brain. Occasionally, migraine aura may persist, giving rise to stroke, a rare condition called 'true migrainous infarction'. There is good evidence that migraine may give rise to stroke. When stroke occurs as an immediate sequela of a migraine attack, only 9% of patients have an arterial lesion; however, if the stroke occurs well after the migraine attack, 91% have an arterial lesion. This indicates that mechanisms other than traditional arterial disease may underlie migrainous infarction.

Migraine is also a risk factor for stroke remote from the migraine, particularly in women under 45 years of age. For women with migraine who smoke or use oral contraceptives, stroke risk is substantially increased. Although the relative risk of stroke in women under 45 years old who have migraine is increased 3- to 4-fold, the absolute risk of stroke remains low. Women with migraine should be advised not to smoke. We consider the risk of oral contraceptives acceptable, although we believe that this issue should be discussed with the patient.

Welch proposed a system to classify migraine-related stroke (Table 3.3). In none of the four categories can a causal attribution between stroke and migraine be made with certainty. For 'coexisting stroke and migraine', the stroke must occur at a time without migraine. This form of migraine-related stroke may sometimes be explained by risk factors associated with both the migraine and stroke, such as mitral valve prolapse. For 'stroke with clinical features of migraine', a clear-cut stroke syndrome gives rise to secondary headaches that resemble migraine. For example, carotid dissection and arteriovenous malformations (AVMs) may mimic migraine. Migraine-induced stroke in Welch's classification is termed 'true migrainous infarction' in the IHS classification. Finally, there is a substantial group of patients whose migraine and stroke occur together, but the relationship is uncertain.

Migraine and epilepsy

Migraine and epilepsy are comorbid. The median prevalence of epilepsy in migraine sufferers across a series of studies is 5.9% (range: 1–17%), which greatly exceeds the prevalence of epilepsy in general populations (0.5%). In a large study, migraine was 2.4 times more common in individuals with epilepsy than in their relatives without epilepsy. Thus, studies of individuals with epilepsy demonstrate an increased risk of migraine, and studies in migraine sufferers demonstrate an increased risk of epilepsy.

Factors that influence the relationship between migraine and epilepsy have been investigated. Migraine risk is equally elevated among patients with partial and generalized seizures, but is highest in those patients with post-traumatic epilepsy (relative risk – 4.1 times). Risk is not related to the age of epilepsy onset. In analyses that consider age of onset, migraine risk is elevated both before and after seizure onset. Therefore, migraine cannot be viewed solely as the cause or the consequence of epilepsy. Neither can environmental risk factors nor shared genetic risk factors fully account for comorbidity. Perhaps an altered brain state characterized by neuronal excitability increases the risk of both migraine and epilepsy and accounts for their comorbidity. Genetic or environmental risk factors may increase neuronal excitability or decrease the threshold for both types of attack. A reduction in brain magnesium or alterations in neurotransmitters provide plausible potential substrates for this postulated alteration in neuronal excitability.

The association between migraine and epilepsy has implications for clinical practice. When treating patients for one disorder, it is important to maintain a heightened index of suspicion for the other disorder. As migraine is more common than epilepsy, this is especially important when treating patients with epilepsy. It can be difficult to differentiate migraine and epilepsy because both conditions are characterized by episodes of neurological dysfunction. The most

● **Table 3.3** *Classification of migraine-related stroke*

Category	Feature
I	Coexisting stroke and migraine

II	Stroke with clinical features of migraine
	  A Symptomatic migraine
	  B Migraine mimic

III	Migraine-induced stroke
	  A Without risk factors
	  B With risk factors

IV	Uncertain

common form of this problem is the differential diagnosis of migraine with aura from partial complex seizure, especially if the attacks are accompanied by perplexity and headache. Epilepsy is more likely if the aura is brief (less than 5 minutes) and associated with alteration of consciousness, automatisms, and other positive motor functions (tonic–clonic movements). Migraine is more likely if the aura lasts longer than 5 minutes and has positive (scintillations, tingling) and negative (visual loss, numbness) features.

Treatment strategies for patients with comorbid migraine and epilepsy need to be governed by their simultaneous presence. For example, in treating migraine, drugs that lower seizure threshold must be used cautiously (these drugs include tricyclic antidepressants, selective serotonin reuptake inhibitors, and neuroleptics). Treating both migraine and epilepsy with a single drug may be advantageous. Sodium valproate has well-established efficacy in this setting.

Migraine, major affective disorders, and anxiety

Recent population-based studies demonstrate an association between migraine and major depression, bipolar disorder, panic disorder, and anxiety disorder. Comorbid psychiatric disease is also apparently associated with seeking care for headache disorders, as indicated by a study that showed a history of panic disorder in an unexpectedly high proportion of those who consulted a physician for headache. In another study, both major depression and anxiety disorders were commonly found in migraineurs. Furthermore, in patients with all three disorders, the onset of anxiety generally precedes the onset of migraine, whereas the onset of major depression usually follows the onset of migraine. A bidirectional influence exists in migraine that is comorbid with depression, which indicates that migraine is neither simply a cause nor simply a consequence of depression. The diagnostic work-up is made with a high index of suspicion for psychiatric disease in migraine and for migraine in psychiatric disease. Treatment can include prophylaxis with antidepressants, tricyclic antidepressants, and serotonin re-uptake inhibitors for depression and anxiety, and valproate for manic-depressive disease.

Migraine and personality characteristics

The relationships between migraine and personality characteristics have been discussed far more often than they have been systematically studied. The idea of a migraine personality first grew out of clinical observations of the highly selected patients seen in subspecialty clinics. Many early authors described migraineurs as perfectionist, rigid, competitive, easily frustrated, and overly sensitive. Studies that use personality scales, such as the Minnesota Multiphasic Personality Inventory, are limited when they compare migraineurs with historical norms rather than with concurrent controls, when they do not use explicit diagnostic criteria for migraine, or when a selection bias is introduced, such as in clinic-based populations. However, in the first (1990) population-based, case–control study of personality in migraine, migraineurs' test scores (using the Eysenck Personality Questionnaire [EPQ]) were higher than those of the controls, indicating that they were more tense, anxious, and depressed than the controls. Women with migraine scored significantly higher than controls on the P scale of the EPQ, which measures psychoticism, indicating that they were more hostile, less interpersonally sensitive, and out of step with their peers. However, even the population-based studies have not generally controlled for drug use, headache frequency, headache-related disability, or major psychiatric disorders, all of which would have an impact on the results.

Social impact of migraine

Migraine is a public health problem of enormous scope that has an impact on the individual sufferer and on society. In North America, South America, and Western Europe, migraine affects about 15–18% of women and 4–6% of men. The American Migraine Study estimates that 23 million United States residents have severe migraine headaches. Of the people who suffer from migraine, 25% have more than four severe attacks a month; 35% experience 1–4 severe attacks a month; and 40% experience less than one severe attack a month. The study also found that more than 85% of women and more than 82% of men with severe migraine had some headache-related disability. About one-third were severely disabled or needed bedrest. In addition to attack-related disability, many migraineurs live in fear between attacks, knowing that at any time an attack could disrupt their ability to work, care for their families, or engage in social activities.

Migraine has an enormous impact on society. A population-based diary study in the United States estimated that people with migraine lose the equivalent of 12 days' work per year as a result of headache. This statistic includes 4.4 days lost through absenteeism and 7.6 days caused by reduced productivity due to headache while at work. In the United States, annual lost productivity because of migraine costs about 13 billion dollars per year. Migraine has a marked impact on healthcare as well. The National Ambulatory Medical Care Survey (1976–77) found that 4% of all visits to physicians' offices (over 10 million visits a year) were for headache. Migraine results in major use of emergency rooms and urgent-care centres, and vast amounts of prescription and over-the-counter medication sales.

Although migraine is often a lifelong disorder, some people experience exacerbations and others experience remissions over time. One study followed children with severe migraine for up to 37 years. Among those followed, 62% experienced complete remissions for more than 2 years. After 30 years of follow-up, 40% were migraine-free, although 60% continued to have migraine. A number of reports suggest that migraine can be a progressive disease. A subgroup of migraineurs are afflicted with a syndrome variously called 'chronic daily headache evolving from migraine', 'transformed migraine', or 'malignant migraine'. In this syndrome, attacks increase in number but decrease in severity over the years until a pattern of daily headache evolves. In headache clinics, about 80% of patients who have daily or near-daily headache overuse acute headache medication, an overuse that contributes to an accelerating pattern of pain through the mechanism of 'rebound headache' (*see* Chapter 8). However, the remaining 20% of patients experience this accelerating pattern of pain even without medication overuse, which suggests that one subgroup of migraineurs worsens progressively. In population studies, 4–5% of the general population experiences headaches 15 or more days per month. This aetiologically heterogeneous 'frequent headache' group is discussed in Chapter 8.

Genetics of migraine

Many studies have examined the transmission of migraine within families, the occurrence of migraine among twins, and the link of migraine to specific chromosomal loci. Migraine recently entered the era of molecular study when researchers found that a genetic locus on chromosome 19, involved in familial hemiplegic migraine (FHM), codes for a specific type of calcium channel subunit.

Studies of family risk of migraine

Controlled studies show that the risk of migraine is increased among the relatives of people with migraine. One recent population-based study indicated that first-degree relatives of migraineurs who have aura have four times the risk of migraine with aura. Relatives of individuals with migraine without aura have 1.9 times the risk of migraine without aura. In this study, transmission of migraine within families appears to be specific as to type. Other population-based studies demonstrate familial aggregation at similar rates but do not confirm that the two forms run within families.

Twin studies

Clinic- and population-based studies show that identical (monozygotic) twins are more likely to have migraine in common than fraternal (dizygotic) twins do. These results support an aetiological role for genetic factors. However, the twin studies also demonstrate that genetic factors cannot fully account for migraine. Identical twins, with 100% of their genes in common, often differ in their migraine status. Thus, the twin studies strongly suggest that genetic factors are important and prove that environmental factors play a role.

Linkage studies

Linkage studies serve to determine patterns of transmission. Efforts are underway to identify specific chromosomal loci and specific migraine genes. As stated above, in FHM, a rare autosomal dominant disorder with hemiplegia as one component of the aura, linkage to chromosome 19 has been demonstrated in about half of the families studied to date. A Dutch research group identified a neuronal calcium channel protein believed to be the product of the pathogenic gene on chromosome 19. Possibly the gene or genes involved in non-chromosome 19 FHM may code for a functionally related protein (*see* Chapter 5). The relationship between this chromosome 19 linkage marker or gene product and more common types of migraine is not yet clear.

Epidemiology of tension-type headache

Recent epidemiological studies provide estimates of the prevalence of tension-type headache. Episodic tension-type headache affects roughly 40% of the population, with a slight female preponderance. Although migraine prevalence is inversely related to socioeconomic status, the prevalence of episodic tension-type headache increases with education. Chronic tension-type headache, characterized by 15 or more attacks per month, has a prevalence of 2–3%, with a greater female preponderance. In population studies, chronic tension-type headache is the most common cause of frequent headache.

Tension-type headache often interferes with activities of daily living. In a given year, about 18% of people with tension-type headache have to discontinue normal activity, while 44% experience some limited function. Attacks occur with a mean frequency of 2.9 days a month or 35 days a year. Most sufferers have fewer than one attack a month, and about one-third have two or more attacks a month. Like migraine, tension-type headache strikes individuals early in life and continues to affect them through their peak productive years. All migraineurs and 60% of people with tension-type headache have a diminished capacity for work and other activities. Despite their disability, about 50% of migraineurs and 80% of people with tension-type headache have not consulted their general practitioner about their headaches at all.

Individuals with frequent episodic tension-type headache may be at increased risk for chronic tension-type headache. Many people with migraine also have attacks of tension-type headache – tension-type headaches occur in individuals with migraine at rates greater than predicted by the coincidental co-occurrence of common disorders in the same individual. Further, tension-type headaches in migraine sufferers show dramatic treatment responses to sumatriptan, while tension-type headaches in isolation do not. Thus, tension-type headache in migraine may be quite different in epidemiology, biology, and treatment than tension-type headache in isolation.

Summary

- Migraine is a highly prevalent disorder that affects 15–18% of women and 6% of men. Since it is most common during the peak productive years (25–55 years of age), it has an enormous impact as measured by lost work and reduced productivity at work.
- Less than half of migraine sufferers have seen a doctor for headache within the past year; many people outside the healthcare system have high levels of pain and disability and would benefit from treatment.
- Migraine is comorbid (more than coincidentally associated) with epilepsy, depression, manic-depressive illness, anxiety disorders, and stroke (among young women). Comorbidity creates a mandate for diagnostic and therapeutic vigilance. Treatment strategies must be governed by the presence of comorbid disease.
- Although migraine is a stroke risk factor in young women, the relationships between migraine and stroke are complex. Stroke may trigger vascular headache, migraine aura may persist in the form of stroke (migrainous infarction), or the association may be modified by underlying factors, such as medication use, mitral valve prolapse, carotid artery disease, etc.
- Although studies that link personality to migraine are difficult to conduct, population-based, case–control studies indicate that migraineurs tend to be more tense, anxious, and depressed than do controls.
- Genetic factors play a critical role in determining the risk of migraine. Pathogenic genes have been identified for one rare form of migraine. Genes for more common forms are being sought.
- Tension-type headache is far more common than migraine, affecting 40% of the general population. Although its burden is less severe than that of migraine for individual headache sufferers, the aggregate social burden is great because the condition is so prevalent.

Further reading

Rasmussen BK. Epidemiology of headache. *Cephalalgia* 1995; 15: 45–68.

Rasmussen BK, Jensen R, Schroll M, Olesen J. Epidemiology of headache in a general population – a prevalence study. *J Clin Epidemiol* 1991; 44: 1147–57.

Rothrock J, North J, Madden K et al. Migraine and migrainous stroke: risk factors and prognosis. *Neurology* 1993; 43: 2473–6.

Steward WF, Lipton RB, Celentano DD, Reed ML. Prevalence of migraine headache in the United States. *JAMA* 1992; 267: 64–9.

Welch KMA, Levin SR. Migraine-related stroke in the context of the IHS classification of migraine. *Arch Neurol* 1990; 49–62.

4 Diagnostic testing and ominous causes of headache

Headache diagnosis is based primarily on a thorough history and physical and neurological examinations. Diagnostic tests should be used selectively when suspicion arises for specific disorders and should be based on a careful clinical assessment. Diagnostic testing (Table 4.1) may:

- identify serious underlying diseases (e.g. neuroimaging may identify stroke, tumour, subdural haematoma, or arteriovenous malformation [AVM]);
- identify associated diseases that could complicate headache and its treatment (e.g. laboratory tests may identify Lyme disease or hypothyroidism);
- establish a baseline for drug treatment (e.g. liver function tests prior to valproate [divalproex] treatment);
- reveal contraindications to drug treatment (e.g. ischaemic changes on electrocardiogram [EKG] prior to triptan therapy); and
- measure drug levels to determine compliance, absorption, or medication overuse.

In addition, diagnostic testing is often recommended to:

- increase diagnostic certainty and relieve the clinician's anxiety;
- address the patient's expectations and concerns;
- provide a shortcut for a thorough evaluation;
- satisfy a referring clinician when tests are expected; and
- provide information in a medical–legal context.

Choosing the appropriate diagnostic tests to perform is often difficult. Few controlled trials or guidelines define which studies are appropriate in which circumstances; however, failing to obtain a necessary test can have grave consequences for both patient and physician. Health plans sometimes limit access to studies, and lack of funds or insurance are barriers to appropriate testing for many patients. To use tests appropriately, it is useful to understand the principles that underlie the evaluation of diagnostic tests, which is their sensitivity and specificity relative to some 'gold standard':

- *sensitivity* is defined according to the proportion of individuals who have a disease and have a positive test result – a test with high sensitivity identifies almost everyone with the disease; and
- *specificity* is the proportion of individuals who do *not* have the disease and have a negative result on the test – if specificity is high, false positive results are few.

In this chapter, we report the sensitivity and specificity of the diagnostic tests discussed when that information is available. Chapter 2 recommends that the clinician search for headache alarms in every patient, based on the history and physical examination (Figure 2.1); if alarms are present, some important considerations in

● **Table 4.1** Why do headache studies?

Study	Diagnosis	Baseline	Compliance/toxicity
Complete blood cell count, differential	✓	✓	✓
Sedimentation rate	✓		
Chemistry profile	✓	✓	✓
Electrocardiogram		✓	✓
Blood gases	✓		
Drug screen	✓		✓
Drug level			✓
Lyme disease, HIV, VDRL	✓		
ANA, lupus anticoagulant, anticardiolipin antibodies	✓		

HIV = human immunodeficiency virus; VDRL = venereal disease research laboratory; ANA = antinuclear antibody.

differential diagnosis are indicated, and methods of work-up are proposed (Table 2.3).

Important headache alarms that suggest the need for diagnostic testing include:

- the first headache in a patient over 50 years of age;
- sudden onset or 'thunderclap' headache;
- marked change in headache pattern (increased frequency, intensity, or duration);
- neurological signs and symptoms other than those of a typical migraine aura (i.e. diplopia, blindness, confusion, dizziness, weakness, sensory loss);
- meningeal signs – neck stiffness, positive Kernig's or Brudzinski's sign;
- unexplained fever;
- persistent or unexplained vomiting;
- recent malignancy, non-trivial head trauma, or convulsions;
- worsening headache; and
- blood pressure higher than 180/115 mmHg.

A number of factors suggest that the headaches are more likely to be primary. The following factors lessen the need to investigate a headache:

- regular or near-regular perimenstrual or periovulatory timing of the headache;
- its appearance after *sustained* exertion;
- its abatement with sleep; and
- food, odour, or weather changes provoking headaches.

Methods of investigation

In a typical healthy migraineur, laboratory tests are not necessary for diagnosis, but may be needed prior to treatment. We routinely obtain an EKG in patients with cardiac risk factors prior to the use of triptans, ergots, or other vasoconstrictors, and we obtain liver function tests prior to the use of valproate. We often obtain a complete blood count (CBC) and chemistry profile before we initiate therapy. The antinuclear antibody test screens for autoimmune conditions. An erythrocyte sedimentation rate not only acts as a screen for serious diseases such as a malignancy or collagen vascular disease, but it can also establish the diagnosis of temporal arteritis, which is a cause of headache in the elderly. Thyroid function studies are performed to rule out thyroid disease, such as thyrotoxicosis, a condition that may exacerbate headache and is a relative contraindication to ergot administration. In addition, we obtain thyroid studies prior to the use of lithium and for patients with comorbid depression. Unexpected or overused medications that have a direct impact on headache and its treatment can be identified by means of drug screening and toxicology studies. Specific studies, such as electrolytes and liver or kidney function tests, may be needed before starting drug treatment. Routine testing for Lyme disease is not recommended. If the headache is atypical or accompanied by systemic or neurological manifestations of Lyme disease, we suggest serum antibody testing by enzyme-linked immunoabsorbent assay (ELISA).

Electroencephalography

Although electroencephalography (EEG) is noninvasive and relatively inexpensive, it is not useful in the routine assessment of headache sufferers. Between 12 and 15% of healthy adults with no history of head injury, seizures, headaches, or other neurological diseases have non-specific EEG abnormalities. The American Academy of Neurology (AAN) reviewed the literature on EEG used to diagnose headache and found many studies that were flawed because of selection methods, lack of controls, or other design problems. Studies designed to determine whether specific groups of headache patients have an increased prevalence of EEG abnormalities have been inconclusive. Since EEG neither adequately screens for structural causes of headache nor differentiates primary headache subgroups, the AAN concluded that EEG is not useful in the routine evaluation of patients presenting only with headache. Indications for EEG in headache investigation are described in Table 4.2.

Computed tomography and magnetic resonance imaging

The AAN reviewed the role of neuroimaging to evaluate headache patients when the neurological examination is normal. Their analysis was

● **Table 4.2** *Indications for ordering EEG*

- Alteration or loss of consciousness
- Transient neurological symptoms without ensuing headache
- Suspected encephalopathy
- Residual persisting neurological defects
- Baseline EEG prior to the institution of medicines or procedures that could induce seizures
- Suspicion of comorbid epilepsy

● **Table 4.4** *Approximate probability of recognizing an aneurysmal subarachnoid hemorrhage on computed tomographic scan after the initial event*

Time after initial event	Probability (%)
Day 0	95
Day 3	74
Week 1	50
Week 2	30
Week 3	Almost 0

From Adams et al., 1983, and VanGijn and VanDongen, 1982

● **Table 4.3** *Indications for neuroimaging*

- The first headache in a patient over 50 years of age
- Sudden onset or 'thunderclap' headache
- Marked change in headache pattern (increased frequency, intensity, or duration)
- Neurological signs and symptoms other than those of a typical migraine aura (i.e. diplopia, blindness, confusion, dizziness, weakness, sensory loss)
- Meningeal signs – neck stiffness, positive Kernig's or Brudzinski's sign
- Recent malignancy, non-trivial head trauma, or convulsions
- Worsening headache

based on 16 studies that used computed tomography (CT) or magnetic resonance imaging (MRI) and mostly comprised retrospective case series. The AAN report concluded that the routine use of CT and MRI is not warranted for patients with recurrent migraine headache if there has been no recent change in the headache pattern, no history of seizures, and no focal neurological findings. Migraineurs have a higher prevalence of non-specific white matter abnormalities on MRI than do non-migraineurs, but these findings cannot be used to diagnose migraine, change treatment, or predict prognosis. Patients with brain tumours can have headaches that resemble migraine or tension-type headache. These headaches are often progressive and of late onset or are associated with seizures, confusion, prolonged nausea, hemiparesis, papilloedema, or other neurological abnormalities. Indications for CT or MRI in headache investigation are described in Table 4.3.

In addition, imaging should be considered for patients whose headaches are atypical and do not fit into any defined primary headache group.

Both CT and MRI have been used in patients with suspected aneurysmal subarachnoid haemorrhage (SAH). As CT scan (without contrast) is very sensitive in the first 24 hours after headache onset it is the neuroimaging modality of choice for detecting acute SAH. Using lumbar puncture (LP) as the gold standard, CT scan can identify subarachnoid blood in 92% of patients with aneurysmal SAH in the first 24 hours; this decreases to 58% by day 5. In one study of SAH, the percentage of scans that were normal in the first 24 hours was 3.3%; on day 1, this increased to 7.2%; and on day 5 to 27.3% (Table 4.4). For detecting SAH, MRI is almost equal to CT during the first 24 hours, slightly superior to CT from 24 to 72 hours, and from 3 to 14 days MRI is superior to CT. Thus, the physician should use CT first for the diagnosis of SAH up to 3 days after onset, and then use MRI.

Cerebral angiography

Unless the physician suspects cerebral aneurysm, vasculitis, or AVM, there is little reason to perform angiography for the evaluation of headache in a patient with a normal neurological examination, a normal CT or MRI, and a history consistent with a benign primary headache disorder. Transient neurological symptoms may occur following cerebral angiography, especially among patients who have migraine with aura.

Magnetic resonance angiography

In spite of its limitations, magnetic resonance angiography (MRA) is a safe and non-invasive tool that is useful for screening for suspected aneurysm or AVM in patients without SAH. Although MRA detects aneurysms as small as 3–4 mm in the circle of Willis, it has the following limitations:

- small aneurysms may be better visualized than larger, thrombosed aneurysms; and
- high signal intensity thrombus within an aneurysm could be mistaken for slow blood flow.

Lumbar puncture

The LP is crucial to diagnosis in four clinical situations:

- first-or-worst headache syndrome;
- severe, rapid-onset, recurrent headache;
- progressive headache; and
- atypical chronic intractable headache.

The physician should perform an LP if neuroimaging is normal, non-diagnostic of the suspected disorder, or suggestive of a disorder that can only be diagnosed by cerebrospinal fluid (CSF) pressure measurement, cell count, and chemistries. The LP is performed first if neuroimaging is not available and meningitis is suspected, especially in the absence of focality or papilloedema on the neurological examination.

The patient who presents with the sudden onset of a 'first-or-worst' headache should be evaluated for an acute neurological event, although the physician should keep in mind that migraine can also present this way. Focal neurological signs or symptoms or a change in consciousness or mental status suggest an intracranial process. Distinguishing between the first severe, acute-onset migraine (crash migraine) and SAH is almost impossible. A brain image should be performed, if possible prior to LP.

An LP is crucial to rule out an intracranial infection in the patient who presents with a confusional state, fever, or meningeal signs (with or without headache). If CT is readily available, it is performed before the LP. However, if an imaging procedure is not readily available, an LP is performed, particularly when the physician suspects meningitis. Delaying the LP delays the diagnosis, and may result in increased morbidity and mortality. If the headache has the characteristics of a postural (orthostatic) headache with no obvious cause (such as a prior diagnostic LP or myelogram), an LP may help establish the diagnosis of low CSF pressure headache.

Many disorders are associated with increased intracranial pressure. Patients with papilloedema and suspected increased intracranial pressure should have a neuroimaging procedure (MRI or CT) to rule out a mass lesion. If these studies are normal, the physician can make a tentative diagnosis of idiopathic intracranial hypertension. However, chronic meningitis can produce increased intracranial pressure, so an LP is crucial to document increased intracranial pressure, rule out chronic meningitis (particularly in patients who are immunosuppressed), and ascertain the therapeutic effect of drugs given to decrease intracranial pressure.

A rare and often overlooked cause of head pain is increased intracranial pressure without papilloedema. For example, patients with intractable chronic daily headache commonly fail to respond to the usual headache treatment, and the physician may assume that their problem is not organic in origin. An LP can aid diagnosis in such patients.

Patients with daily headaches of subacute onset can have chronic fungal meningitis (particularly those who are immunosuppressed), the meningitis of Lyme disease, or carcinomatous meningitis, all of which require LP to diagnose. The physician should be aware that CSF pleocytosis occurs rarely in migraine with or without aura. Unless the physician suspects meningitis, SAH, or high- or low-pressure syndrome, LP is not needed during a headache.

Thermography

Thermography does not provide sufficiently reliable information to be useful as a diagnostic test, according to an analysis of the literature by the AAN. Research continues on thermography, with some studies describing abnormal thermograms in headache patients (e.g. temperature asymmetry in migraineurs or a cold spot along the supraorbital area or the inner orbit and canthus in patients with cluster headache and chronic paroxysmal hemicrania).

Electromyography

Electromyography (EMG) does not have sufficient sensitivity or specificity to be useful as a diagnostic test in headache. Some migraine or tension-type headache patients have increased activity in the muscles of the neck and scalp, but no correlation has been shown between increased EMG activity and pain or tenderness.

Investigating specific headache types

Migrainous infarction and migraine with prolonged or atypical aura

The physician should consider the possibility of an organic problem when a migraineur presents with weakness, numbness, speech difficulty, or a persistent visual field defect. The primary care physician should consider a neurological consultation to evaluate for potential stroke, tumour, or subdural haematoma. The patient should undergo MRA or arteriography promptly if carotid disease, vasculitis, or large artery dissection is suspected. Other tests that may also be necessary to look for a cause of the stroke are carotid duplex scanning (echo), transcranial Doppler, electrocardiogram, and Holter monitoring. For patients under 55 years of age, antiphospholipid antibodies, protein S, protein C, and occasionally antithrombin III levels may need to be determined when the cause of stroke is not obvious. These are recently discovered contributing factors to stroke that act to enhance coagulability.

Basilar migraine

Another cause of neurological symptoms is basilar migraine, described in Chapter 6. When a patient has syncope, diplopia, vertigo, ataxia, a change in mental state, and confusion, the physician should suspect basilar migraine and seek neurological consultation. The consultant may order an EEG to determine whether epileptiform activity is present and MRI or CT to exclude a space-occupying lesion or a brainstem AVM. If vertebrobasilar disease is suspected, especially in older patients, MRA and transcranial Doppler are indicated. In some cases, if the physician is uncertain whether vascular disease is present, an angiogram may be necessary.

Migraine aura without headache

Diagnostic criteria for migraine aura without headache (late life migrainous equivalents) are outlined in Table 4.5. When a patient has a migraine-like aura with mild headache or no headache at all, it may be difficult to differentiate

● **Table 4.5** *Late-life migrainous equivalents*

- The gradual appearance of focal neurological symptoms, spreading or intensifying over a period of minutes, not seconds
- Positive visual symptoms characteristic of 'classic' migraine, even if these come on abruptly, specifically fortification spectra (scintillating scotoma), flashing lights, dazzles, or a 'march' of paraesthesias
- Previous similar symptoms associated with 'classic' migraine or a more severe headache
- Serial progression from one accompaniment to another, such as a visual aura progressing to an aura with paraesthesias
- The occurrence of two or more identical spells
- A duration of 15–25 minutes (transient ischaemic attacks usually last less than 15 minutes)
- The occurrence of a 'flurry' of accompaniments (these generally occur in the 50–60-year-old age group)
- A generally benign course without permanent sequelae

migraine from a transient ischaemic attack (TIA) without using neuroimaging and arteriograms, and neurological consultation may be needed. Conditions that need to be excluded are cerebral thrombosis, embolism, dissection, subclavian steal syndrome, epilepsy, thrombocytopenia, polycythaemia, hyperviscosity syndrome, and antiphospholipid antibody syndrome.

The symptoms of migraine aura without headache are usually visual and are often bilateral (71% of cases) and associated with other aura symptoms (sensory disturbances, aphasia, or dysarthria), unlike TIA symptoms, which seem to be one-sided and non-visual. Attacks of migraine aura without headache are typically longer in duration than are TIAs, lasting between 15 and 60 minutes. If the symptoms are bilateral or not visual, a neurological consultation should be considered.

The manifestations of migraine aura without headache vary in extent, duration, severity, and quality. Diagnosis is more difficult when the condition occurs for the first time in a patient over 40 years of age unless classic symptoms, such as a scintillating scotoma, are present.

Headache of sudden onset

A headache that has a sudden onset and extended duration may indicate a SAH or might be a warning (sentinel headache) of a future major SAH. More benign causes of headache of

● **Table 4.6** Headache of sudden onset

Primary headache disorders
- Crash migraine
- Cluster
- Benign exertional headache
- Benign orgasmic cephalgia

Secondary headache disorders
- Associated with vascular disorders
  Unruptured saccular aneurysm
  Subarachnoid haemorrhage
  Internal carotid artery dissection
  Cerebral venous thrombosis
  Acute hypertension
    pressor response
    phaeochromocytoma
- Associated with non-vascular intracranial disorders
  Intermittent hydrocephalus
  Benign intracranial hypertension
  Pituitary apoplexy
  Cephalic infection
    meningoencephalitis
    acute sinusitis
  Acute mountain sickness
  Disorders of eyes
    acute optic neuritis
    acute glaucoma

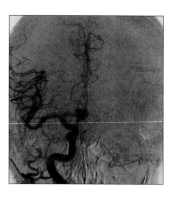

● **Figure 4.1**
Unruptured
aneurysms.

ing CT and LP, is indicated. Of the diagnostic tests, only LP can unerringly diagnose SAH. A CT can miss 25% of SAH, particularly if the CT is not carried out until days after the headache onset. After 24 hours, MRI may be more sensitive than CT. The frequency of unruptured aneurysm among patients with thunderclap headache is unknown. Patients with unruptured aneurysms can present with ocular palsy, thunderclap headache, or even seizures. Often the CT and LP are normal and consultation is indicated. Most, but not all, experts now believe that all patients in whom unruptured aneurysm is a possibility should undergo an MRA at the least. The routine use of cerebral angiography is proscribed by the risk of permanent (0.1%) and transient (1.2%) deficits in this low-yield population (Figure 4.1).

Coital headache

Several headache types are associated with sexual activity (Table 4.7). Coital headache pain, which usually begins at or shortly before orgasm, is intense, located in the frontal or occipital area, is explosive or throbbing, and persists for a few minutes to 48 hours. This manifestation can be ominous and suggestive of an SAH. A CT should be performed, and even if the findings are negative, an LP should be obtained. Another less ominous type of coital headache begins earlier in intercourse, has an occipital or diffuse location, and a dull and aching pain that is most severe at orgasm. Benign sexual headache occurs earlier in life than the symptomatic variety and is often associated with exertional headache.

Exertional and cough headaches

Coughing and exertion can aggravate any headache or (rarely) provoke a new headache.

sudden onset include migraine of sudden onset ('crash migraine') and coital cephalgia (Table 4.6). A severe headache of sudden onset that reaches maximum intensity within 1 minute is often referred to as a thunderclap headache.

The classic presentation of SAH caused by a ruptured aneurysm includes acute-onset, severe headache associated with a stiff neck, photophobia, nausea, vomiting, and perhaps decreased consciousness or coma. If it presents with this catastrophic picture, SAH is easily differentiated from migraine, but it is often preceded by a minor haemorrhage (which can occur weeks before) that can produce a sentinel headache and be a warning sign of a major rupture.

The first or worst attack of migraine may be difficult to differentiate from SAH, particularly if the pain is rapid in onset. If the patient presents with a first or thunderclap headache associated with focal neurological signs, stiff neck, or changes in cognition, an extensive neurological evaluation, includ-

● **Table 4.7** *International Headache Society diagnostic criteria for coital headache*

4.6 Headache associated with sexual activity

A	Precipitated by sexual excitement
B	Bilateral in onset
C	Prevented or eased by ceasing sexual activity before orgasm
D	Not associated with an intracranial disorder such as aneurysm

● **Table 4.8** *Causes of brief severe headache*

Bilateral	Unilateral
Idiopathic, stabbing headache	Idiopathic stabbing headache
Benign cough and exertional headache	Trigeminal neuralgia
Coital headache	SUNCT
Headaches due to structural disease	Chronic and episodic paroxysmal hemicrania
Colloid cyst of IIIrd ventricle and other IIIrd ventricular tumours	Cluster headache
Pineal region tumours and masses	
Arnold–Chiari malformation	
Platybasia/basilar impression	
Phaeochromocytoma	

SUNCT = short-lasting unilateral neuralgiform headache with conjunctival injection and tearing.

This headache can be symptomatic of an intracranial disorder or it can be an unpleasant but harmless inconvenience. Benign cough headache is a bilateral headache of sudden onset that is precipitated by coughing and lasts less than 1 minute. Benign exertional headache is a bilateral, throbbing headache that lasts from 5 minutes to 24 hours. It is specifically provoked by physical exercise. Neither of these headaches is associated with any systemic or intracranial disorder.

In a recent study, symptomatic cough headache cases were more frequent than benign headache cases (57% versus 43%). Symptomatic cough headaches begin earlier in life and last longer than benign cough headaches. All the patients in the series who had symptomatic cough headache developed posterior fossa manifestations. The benign cough headaches were relieved by indomethacin, but the symptomatic cough headaches were not. Three patients who initially had isolated cough headache and did not respond to indomethacin underwent MRI that demonstrated tonsillar descent. Since MRI was not performed in all benign cough headache patients in this series, some could have had tonsillar descent.

In cough headache MRI must be performed to rule out hindbrain abnormalities, including Arnold–Chiari malformation, posterior fossa meningioma, midbrain cyst, basilar impression, and acoustic neuroma.

Symptomatic exertional headaches begin later in life and last longer than benign exertional headaches. Male predominance was not present in the symptomatic exertional headache group. All patients with symptomatic headaches had manifestations of meningeal irritation or intracra-

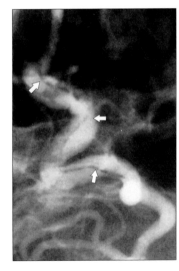

● **Figure 4.2** *Internal carotid artery dissection. (Reproduced with permission from Mokri B et al., 1997.)*

nial hypertension. Those with subarachnoid bleeding had only one headache episode. Neuroradiological evaluation does not need to be carried out for patients with clinical benign sexual or exertional headaches (men around the third decade of life, with a normal examination and short-duration, multiple episodes of pulsating pain that responds to ergotamine or to preventive beta-blockers). The remaining patients must have brain CT and CSF examination if the CT scan is normal. Other causes of brief headache are listed in Table 4.8.

Spontaneous internal carotid artery dissection

Spontaneous internal carotid artery (ICA) dissection is an uncommon cause of headache, but a more common cause of acute neurological deficit in younger patients. The most common symptom, headache, is often unilateral and located in the orbital, periorbital, and frontal regions. The pain is usually moderate to severe, steady or throbbing, and often accompanied by neck pain. A bruit or Horner's syndrome (the association of a small pupil and ptosis) is often present. Focal cerebral symptoms, such as those of TIA or stroke, may precede the headache or follow it within 2 weeks. The gold standard test for spontaneous ICA dissection is arteriography. High-resolution MRI and MRA are being used more often to diagnose ICA dissection because they demonstrate the vessel lumina and changes in the arterial wall (Figure 4.2).

Summary

- Diagnostic tests can help to exclude organic causes of headache, identify comorbid disease, and determine appropriate treatment.
- EEG, thermography, and EMG do not help in the routine evaluation of recurrent headache in the absence of specific indications.
- LP is crucial to diagnose patients who present with their first or worst headache; severe, rapid-onset headache; progressively worsening headache; atypical chronic intractable headache; or headache accompanied by fever and stiff neck.
- Neuroimaging is not routinely indicated in adult patients with recurrent headaches that meet the criteria for migraine or episodic tension-type headache. Neuroimaging should be considered if headache alarms are present, the headache pattern has changed, or focal findings or seizures occur.
- Specific testing (MRI, CT, or LP) is appropriate prior to beginning treatment if the patient is at risk, the treatment poses a risk, or worrisome clinical features are present.
- Consultation and additional testing are often indicated for patients with thunderclap headache, chronic daily headache, headache associated with focal neurological signs, fever, nuchal rigidity, or headache beginning after 55 years of age.

Further reading

Adams HP, Kassell NF, Torner JC, Sahs AL. CT and clinical correlations in recent aneurysmal subarachnoid hemorrhage: a preliminary report of the cooperative aneurysm study. *Neurology* 1983; 33: 981–8.

Evans RW. Diagnostic testing for the evaluation of headaches. *Neurol Clin* 1996; 14: 1–26.

Frishberg BM. The utility of neuroimaging in the evaluation of headache in patients with normal neurologic examinations. *Neurology* 1994; 44: 1191–7.

Harling DW, Peatfield RC, Van Hille PT, Abbott RJ. Thunderclap headache: is it migraine? *Cephalalgia* 1989; 9: 87–90.

Lance JW, Goadsby PJ. *Mechanism and Management of Headache*, 6th edn. London: Butterworth–Heinemann, 1998.

Mokri B. Headache in spontaneous carotid and vertebral artery dissections. In: Goadsby PJ, Silberstein SD (eds). *Headache*. Boston: Butterworth–Heinemann, 1997: 327–54.

Pascual J, Igelsias F, Oterino A, Vazquez-Barquero A, Berciano J. Cough, exertional, and sexual headaches: an analysis of 72 benign and symptomatic cases. *Neurology* 1996; 46: 1520–4.

Report of the Quality Standards Subcommittee of the American Academy of Neurology. Practice parameter: the electroencephalogram in the evaluation of headache (summary statement). *Neurology* 1995; 45: 1411–13.

Silberstein SD. Evaluation and emergency treatment of headache. *Headache* 1992; 32(8): 396–407.

VanGijn J, VanDongen KG. The time course of aneurysmal hemorrhage on computed tomograms. *Neuroradiology* 1982; 23: 153–6.

5 The pathophysiology of primary headache

Headache is a common human experience, diverse in its expression, complex in its manifestation, and somewhat difficult to understand. While the biology may seem daunting, some important common threads can aid understanding and be rewarded by more satisfying clinical interactions. Patients value an explanation of their symptoms, and knowledge of the basic biology facilitates this process. The basic anatomy of the pathways responsible for head pain applies to most manifestations of the problem, independent of the cause. Pain-control systems modulate headaches of all types, independent of cause, and may be primarily involved in some headache syndromes. In this chapter, common themes are presented, as illustrated by migraine, although much of the fundamental anatomy and physiology has implications for all primary headaches. Our current view of migraine is that it is an inherited instability in sensory control systems in the brain. When these systems malfunction, from either an accumulation of triggers or other unidentified mechanisms, the result is pain, gastrointestinal upset, and afferent dysfunction, such as photophobia, phonophobia, and sensitivity to head movement.

Genetics and the state of the brain

Migraine is predominantly an affliction of young people. The strong family association and early onset suggest an important genetic component. Further supporting this likelihood, the first genetic locus for a migrainous disease (familial hemiplegic migraine) was found on chromosome 19p13 (Figure 5.1) to arise from mutations in voltage-gated calcium channels.

This discovery is the beginning of a large effort to unravel the fundamental defects that lead to migraine. The genetic research into the cause of migraine suggests that it results from disease processes that involve ion channel dysfunction,

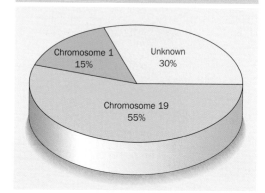

CHROMOSOMAL ALLOCATION OF GENES FOR FAMILIAL HEMIPLEGIC MIGRAINE

Chromosome 1 15%
Unknown 30%
Chromosome 19 55%

● **Figure 5.1** *Chromosomal allocation of genes for familial hemiplegic migraine. About 55% of families can be located on chromosome 19 and 15% on chromosome 1, with the remaining 30% unaccounted for at the present. (Ducros et al., 1997; Gardner et al., 1997 Ophoff et al., 1996.)*

called channelopathies. For example, dysfunction of the calcium channel that mediates 5-hydroxytryptamine (5-HT) release may predispose patients to migraine attacks or impair their self-aborting mechanism. In this context, it is interesting that a magnesium deficiency might be present in the cortex of migraineurs, since magnesium interacts with calcium channels to gate their activation. Calcium channels are also important in the phenomenon of 'spreading depression', which is generally thought to be the basis for the migraine aura.

Spreading depression is a slowly moving wave of neuronal excitation that travels over the cortex, leaving behind suppression of cortical activity. This phenomenon can explain the expanding scintillation of the visual aura (cortical excitation), which is followed by a growing black area of loss of vision, or scotoma (cortical suppression), that is left behind (Figure 5.2). Migraine may also be associated with a state of neuronal hyperexcitability that involves the excitatory amino acid glutamate, and this hyperexcitability may be influenced by low levels of magnesium in the brain.

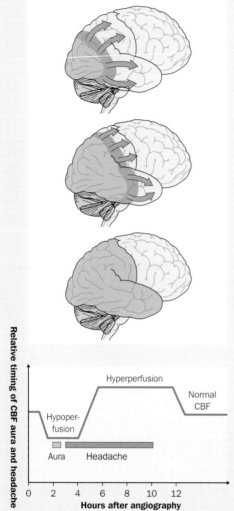

HEADACHE AND CEREBRAL BLOOD FLOW

● **Figure 5.2** *Spreading oligemia observed with studies of cerebral blood flow during aura after Lauritzen (1994).*

Triggers

Triggers can bring on an attack if an individual has increased susceptibility, which may be the core of the basic neurobiology of migraine. This susceptibility or vulnerability is not static, so trigger factors have variable effects in an individual. Migraine sufferers are more sensitive to many things, and their tolerance to change, such as a missed meal, more

sleep than usual, or increased stress, is impaired. Most influences on migraine, including female predominance and the association with menstruation, do not help to identify the site of the problem. Hormonal changes could act to further lower the threshold to migraine from a clinical perspective by either neural or vascular structures. Patients can control their migraine by reducing change, especially when they feel susceptible to an attack.

Migraine: a sum of the parts

Migraine is a syndrome that is most easily recognized when all the parts are present, but it is no less debilitating or less valid if only one element predominates. Migraine attacks may be divided into three essential components: the beginning, the attack, and the resolution. From a biological point of view, how the attack starts and how it stops are the most interesting and the least understood parts. For the sufferer, however, the actual attack is the most important component and, as a result of better understanding, it is becoming more adequately managed. Some of the questions to be examined include:

- Does the brain institute a process to terminate the attack as soon as it starts?
- Are the premonitory features and the aura mechanistically similar?
- What is the basis for the pain?

Stage 1: premonitory features of migraine – the attack begins

About 25% of patients report symptoms of elation, irritability, depression, hunger, thirst, or drowsiness during the 24 hours that precede the headache. These manifestations suggest a hypothalamic site for their origin. Since neurons in the region of the hypothalamus also generate circadian rhythms, they may play a role in the periodicity that is such an important clinical feature of migraine. When premonitory symptoms are understood, the genesis of attacks will become much clearer and we will be better equiped to develop preventative medications and advise patients.

LASHLEY'S AURA

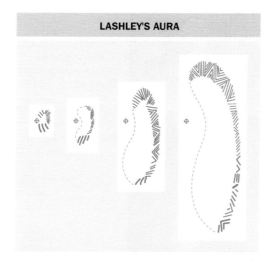

● **Figure 5.3** *Classic illustration of Lashley's aura (1941).*

Stage 2a: the attack – migraine aura

Most patients do not have an aura, but these visual disturbances, such as scintillating scotomata or flashing lights that move across the visual field, are dramatic and have inspired much research (Figure 5.3).

Most clinicians believe that the migraine aura results from neuronal dysfunction, not ischaemia, and that ischaemia rarely, if ever, occurs during the aura. Migraine aura, nevertheless, is associated with reduced cerebral blood flow (CBF; oligaemia) that moves characteristically slowly across the cortex at a rate of 2–3 mm/minute (Figure 5.4). Usually, CBF

changes begin in the occipital region, then may involve the entire hemisphere. Vasoconstriction is not the cause of this reduced blood flow; rather, with reduced neuronal activity, the need for energy and thus CBF is lowered (Figure 5.5). Thus, blood flow follows neuronal activity and the vascular changes are secondary. An important general principle is that both migraine and cluster headache are *neurovascular headaches* – fundamentally nerves drive these diseases and their clinical manifestations.

Once the oligaemia has run its course, blood vessels do not dilate as the result of a normal response to a high carbon dioxide level, but they do respond to changes in blood pressure. This pattern is also seen in spreading depression in experimental studies. A number of studies of migraine patients using single-photon emission computed tomography (SPECT), positron emission tomography (PET), and magnetoencephalography to record CBF or surrogates of neuronal change indicate that spreading oligaemia can occur, yet be clinically silent. Thus, blood flow changes may occur in migraine with and without aura, and this issue is the subject of current work in the field.

Stage 2b: the headache

Anatomy
The trigeminal innervation of pain-producing intracranial structures
A network of mostly unmyelinated fibres arises from the trigeminal ganglion and surrounds the

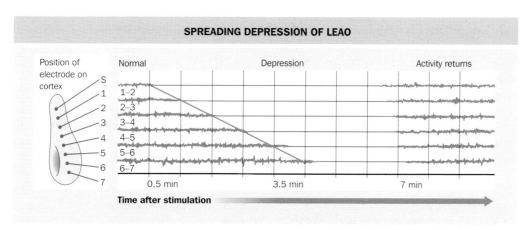

● **Figure 5.4** *Recordings from the rabbit cortex illustrating spreading depression of EEG activity. (Adapted with permission from Leao, 1944.)*

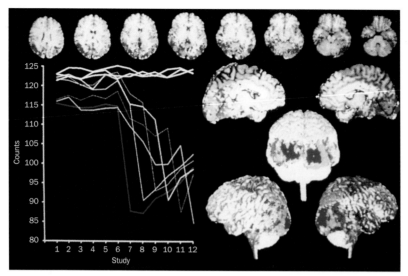

● **Figure 5.5**
Spreading oligaemia demonstrated with positron emission tomography in a young female with a spontaneous attack of migraine. (Reproduced with permission from Woods et al., 1994.)

large cerebral vessels, pial vessels, large venous sinuses, and dura mater. In the posterior fossa, this network arises from the upper cervical dorsal roots. Fibres innervating cerebral vessels arise from within the trigeminal ganglion from neurons that contain neuropeptides (substance P, calcitonin gene-related peptide [CGRP], and neurokinin A) that are released when the trigeminal ganglion is stimulated. Stimulation of the intracranial structures innervated by these fibres, such as the large cerebral vessels and dura mater, produces pain in humans, whereas stimulation of the brain substance itself does not.

Physiology

Potential sources of pain in migraine

Vasoconstriction

Many theories about the cause of migraine have been studied. Harold G. Wolff believed that intracerebral vasoconstriction caused migraine and reactive vasodilation of the carotid artery caused head pain. This explained the throbbing quality of the pain, its varied localization, and its relief by administration of the vasoconstrictor drug, ergotamine. However, the vascular theory runs into difficulty because:

- it does not explain the premonitory features of a migraine attack;
- it does not explain the associated neurological features;

- some of the drugs used to treat migraine have no effect on blood vessels;
- evidence from recent blood flow studies does not support the theory; and
- most patients do not have aura, the initial hypothesized vasoconstrictor phase.

Vasodilation

Dilation of the large intracerebral arteries has been studied as a possible cause of migraine. Two-thirds of migraineurs experience relief if the carotid artery is occluded on the headache side, but one-third do not. Middle cerebral artery dilation, as measured by transcranial Doppler, has been observed during a migraine attack, but no clear relationship exists between control of the headache and subsequent changes in vessel diameter. Moreover, studies show that the oligaemic phase of migraine associated with the aura persists well into the headache phase; thus, migraine headache is not caused simply by cerebrovascular dilation.

Plasma protein extravasation

Sterile neurogenic inflammation has been studied as a possible cause of migraine (Figure 5.6). Stimulation of the trigeminal nerve releases neuropeptides (substance P, CGRP, and neurokinin A), which interact with the blood vessel wall. This produces dilation and capillary leakage of plasma proteins (extravasation), and is a form of sterile inflammation. Electron micrographs show platelet activation in the interior of these

NEURALLY-INDUCED PLASMA PROTEIN EXTRAVASATION MODEL SYSTEM FOR MIGRAINE

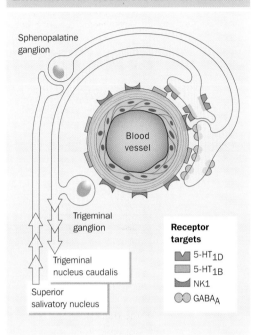

● **Figure 5.6** *Neurally-induced plasma protein extravasation model system for migraine. (Adapted with permission from Cutrer et al., 1997.) NK1: Neurokinin 1, GABA_A: Gamma-aminobutyric acid.*

SENSITIZATION OF MENINGEAL AFFERENTS

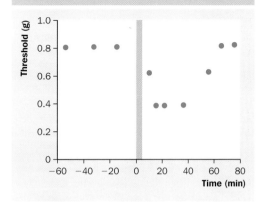

● **Figure 5.7** *Sensitization of primary afferents to mechanical stimulation after application of an inflammatory 'soup'. (Adapted with permission from Strassman et al., 1996.)*

NEUROPEPTIDE CHANGES AND MIGRAINE

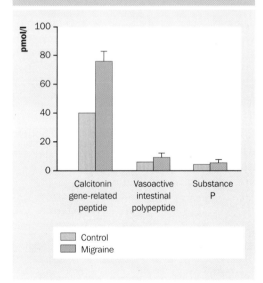

● **Figure 5.8** *Release of vasoactive peptides during migraine. Calcitonin gene-related peptide acts as a marker of trigeminovascular activation during migraine. (Adapted with permission from Edvinsson and Goadsby, 1998.)*

blood vessels that may account for the platelet activation observed during migraine. The sterile inflammatory process is also thought to sensitize nerve fibres to previously innocuous stimuli, such as blood vessel pulsations (Figure 5.7). Sumatriptan, dihydroergotamine, and the newer 5-HT$_{1B/1D}$ agonists, such as eletriptan, naratriptan, rizatriptan, and zolmitriptan, block the release of the neuropeptide and prevent albumin leakage.

Neuropeptides and headache

Levels of CGRP, which is released by the terminals of the trigeminal nerve, rise in animals and humans when the trigeminal ganglion is stimulated. Also, CGRP is released when pain-producing intracranial structures, such as the superior sagittal sinus, are stimulated. During migraine, CGRP is elevated in external jugular venous blood. Such data demonstrate that trigeminovascular neurons are activated during migraine with or without aura, and that treatment with sumatriptan reduces CGRP levels in humans as their migraine subsides (Figure 5.8). In other types of headache, specifically cluster headache and paroxysmal hemicrania (*see* Chapter 9), vasoactive intestinal polypeptide (VIP), a marker for cranial parasympathetic nerve activation, is also elevated. This peptide release offers the prospect of a marker for migraine that can be measured in a venous blood sample and may be helpful in predicting the treatment outcome of medications designed to abort acute migraine attacks.

Central pain processing of trigeminovascular pain

The brainstem sites responsible for craniovascular pain are being mapped using fos-immunohistochemistry, a method for looking at activated cells by imaging a protein that is synthesized when the cells are stimulated. Research data indicate that the trigeminal nucleus cells involved in head pain extend beyond the traditional nucleus caudalis to the dorsal horn of the high cervical region in a functional continuum that could be called *trigeminal nucleus cervicalis*. More than likely, this group of cells, the trigeminocervical neurons (Figure 5.9), is the site for referral of head pain. This anatomical arrangement accounts for the pain distribution found in migraine and other forms of headache and for the referral of pain to both the front and the back of the head.

Information is transmitted to the trigeminocervical neurons in the caudal brainstem and high cervical spinal cord and then relayed to the thalamus. The thalamus passes information on to the cortex. Pain localization may occur in the somatosensory cortex, and emotional or affective responses probably occur in the frontal cortex, anterior cingulate, and insula cortex. Table 5.1 summarizes what is known about the structures that process craniovascular pain.

Stage 3: central modulation – starting and stopping headache

Recent studies reporting brainstem activation in spontaneous migraine attacks emphasize the importance of brainstem mechanisms in the pathogenesis of migraine. In one study, using PET to measure regional CBF (rCBF), nine patients with right-sided migraine without aura were studied within hours of migraine onset. High rCBF values were found bilaterally in the cingulate and in the auditory and visual association cortices. The left side of the brainstem also showed increased rCBF. Sumatriptan relieved the headache and associated symptoms and reversed the cortical

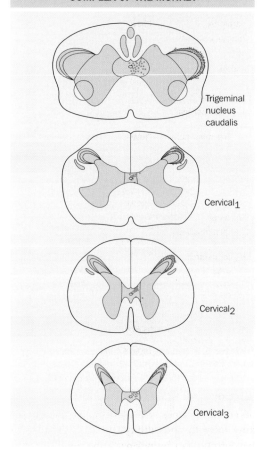

FOS ACTIVATION IN THE TRIGEMINOCERVICAL COMPLEX OF THE MONKEY

Trigeminal nucleus caudalis

Cervical₁

Cervical₂

Cervical₃

● *Figure 5.9* Fos expression (red region) marking the trigeminocervical complex of the monkey. This structure, which extends well into the high cervical spinal cord, is likely to be the anatomical basis for the patterns of head pain seen in most forms of headache. (Adapted with permission from Goadsby and Hoskin, 1997.)

changes, but not the increase in rCBF in the brainstem. Since the increased brainstem rCBF persisted despite headache resolution, it seems likely that the activation results from factors other than, or added to, increased activity of the endogenous pain control (antinociceptive) system. Activation of the brainstem may be inherent in the migraine process itself, marking either a generator or a response system, so that this study may actually be showing us the areas that either start or stop magraine. Continued activation despite symptom resolution with sumatriptan may account for headache recurrence (Figure 5.10).

Table 5.1 *Basic neurobiology of pain-processing in neurovascular headache**

Structure	Pharmacology
Cranial vessels	Serotonin1B (5-HT$_{1B}$)
	Calcitonin gene-related peptide
Trigeminal nerve	5-HT$_{1D}$
	?5-HT$_{1F}$
Dura mater	
Trigeminocervical	
complex	
Trigeminal nerve	Presynaptic 5-HT$_{1D}$
	Postsynaptic N-Methyl-D-aspartate
	α-Amino-3-hydroxy-5-methylisoxa-
	zole-4-proprionic acid
	?Calcitonin gene-related peptide
	?Neurokinin A
Thalamus	
Quintothalamic	?
tract	
Higher centres	
Cingulate cortex	
Insula	
Basal ganglia	
Frontal cortex	?

*Entries based on reasonable evidence from both animal and human studies.

Migraine and the blood–brain barrier

Some compelling data from a clinical study of aura raise the possibility that the blood–brain barrier may not be normal in migraineurs. In a well-conducted study of patients with migraine with aura, the effect of sumatriptan on the aura was examined. Sumatriptan did not change the duration of the aura when compared with placebo. The most fascinating aspect of the study was that sumatriptan was not more effective than placebo for headache when it was given during the aura. However, the headache that continued to develop responded to a second sumatriptan injection. Other studies have shown that treatment failure is associated with the early use of subcutaneous sumatriptan or oral electriptan, which suggests that some process must take hold that facilitates the action of triptans. Triptans may not have access to a crucial receptor site during the aura. The interaction of the drug at its receptor depends on its concentration and its access to the appropriate site, both of which are required to terminate the migraine attack.

Since it is likely that sumatriptan cannot access a site behind the blood–brain barrier, it is possible that the migraineur's blood–brain barrier may not be normal in the headache phase of migraine. Better access to sites within the central nervous system (CNS) may be an advantage in drug development, rather than a drawback. The newer agents all have better access to the CNS and some particular benefits that may relate, in part, to this access.

Central modulation of trigeminovascular pain – the link

Careful study of nerve and brain activation and the changes in CBF that occur during migraine indicates that migraine is most likely a disorder of the CNS. The areas that are active in PET studies

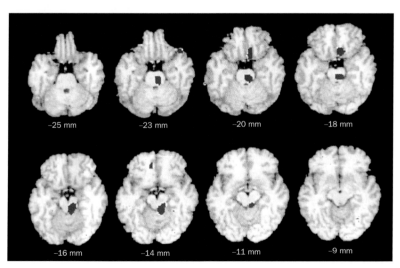

Figure 5.10
Activation of the brainstem with positron emission tomography during acute migraine. (Reproduced with permission from Weiller et al., 1995.)

-25 mm   -23 mm   -20 mm   -18 mm

-16 mm   -14 mm   -11 mm   -9 mm

(Figure 5.10) involve aminergic nuclei that are capable of or involved in:

- altering brain blood flow;
- influencing blood–brain barrier permeability;
- controlling pain information, such as that coming from the trigeminal system; and
- inducing sleep (which is often an excellent way to stop migraine).

Thus, the overall link in the chain of events observed in migraine may be found in the aminergic nuclei in the brainstem. Stimulation of the locus coeruleus, the main noradrenaline-containing cell group in the CNS, can alter brain blood flow and blood–brain barrier permeability. In experimental animals, tricyclic antidepressants alter the blood–brain barrier by modulating the central noradrenergic systems. Central noradrenergic innervation is essential to maintain blood–brain barrier integrity during some pathophysiological states. Moreover, these neurons are involved in controlling sensory signal-to-noise functions that allow animals to attend to information of interest. Many patients note that their concentration is clouded and mention that their brain does not seem *right*. The raphe nuclei, in the midbrain, contain most of the brain serotonin and can influence brain blood flow and gate pain in the thalamus, and also play a role in sleep induction. Migraine may well be a disturbance of the normal interaction between these amine-containing control systems in the brainstem, episodic in its manifestations on the basis of channel dysfunction, described in the section above on genetics (Figure 5.11).

Neuropharmacology of migraine treatment: what can we learn?

Understanding the pathophysiology, biochemistry, and molecular biology of migraine is critical to developing and refining therapeutic solutions to headache. We have learned much from the development of the triptan class of compounds, which are discussed in Chapter 6.

Serotonin and migraine

Strong evidence links migraine and serotonin, which is a central neurotransmitter and vasoconstrictor.

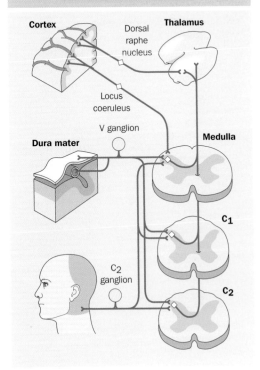

PAIN PROCESSING AND MECHANISMS AND BRAINSTEM CONTROL

● **Figure 5.11** *The essential connections of the trigeminovascular system with the trigeminocervical complex and the brainstem control system. Information from anterior intracranial structures, the dura mater, and the blood vessels projects to the superficial dorsal lamina of the trigeminal nucleus caudalis and the C_1/C_2 cervical spinal cord, the trigeminocervical complex. Projections from branches of C_2 that innervate infratentorial structures synapse on the same neurons; this accounts for referred pain in primary headache syndromes. The information ascends in the quintothalamic tract, synapsing in the contralateral ventrobasal and medial thalamus before projecting to cortex. Aminergic areas in the periaqueductal grey matter (dorsal raphe nucleus) and dorsolateral pontine tegmentum (locus coeruleus) have effects on incoming pain and cortical blood flow. In essence, migraine is an inherited instability in this control system.*

Serotonergic drugs, such as reserpine and *m*-chlorophenylpiperazine, can trigger headaches that are similar to migraine. Depletion of serotonin can induce a migraine attack, while intravenous 5-HT can abort an acute migraine attack. The discovery that 5-HT is responsible for selective cranial vasoconstriction led to the development of sumatriptan.

● **Table 5.2** Classification of serotonin (5-HT) receptors

5-HT receptor class	Second messenger	Antagonist	Function
1	↓Adenylate cyclase		See Table 5.3 for details
2	↑Phosphoino-sitide turnover	Methysergide	Contraction of smooth muscle
		Pizotifen	Central nervous system excitation Subtypes: 2A, 2B, 2C
3	K+ Ca2+ Na+	Ondansetron Granisetron	Membrane depolarization
4	↑Adenylate cyclase	GR113808	Stimulates gastrointestinal contraction Found in striatonigral system
5		—	Subclasses a & b
6		—	Single receptor
7	↑Adenylate cyclase	—	Splice variables Role in circadian rhythms

Modified from Hoyer et al. 1994.

● **Table 5.3** Classification of serotonin (5-HT) subclass 1 receptors.*

Subtype of 5-HT$_1$ receptor	Agonist	Antagonist	Function
A	8-OH-DPAT* Dihydroergo-tamine Sumatriptan Eletriptan Naratriptan Frovatriptan	WAY100165*	Hypotension Behavioural (satiety)
Rat B Human B (previously known as 1$_{D\beta}$)	CP-93,129* Sumatriptan Dihydroergo-tamine Triptans†	GR127935*	Central autoreceptor (rat) Craniovascular receptor
D (previously known as 1$_{D\alpha}$)	Sumatriptan Dihydroergo-tamine Triptans†	GR127935*	Trigeminal Neuronal receptor
E	Dihydroergo-tamine Eletriptan Naratriptan	—	?
F	Sumatriptan Eletriptan Frovatriptan Naratriptan Zolmitriptan LY334370‡	—	?

Modified from Goadsby, 1998.
8-OH-DPAT [8-hydroxy-2-(di-n-propylamino)tetralin], WAY100165, CP-93,129 and GR127935 are compounds used in the laboratory for pharmacological purposes and have no current clinical indications.
†*Triptans: almotriptan, eletriptan, frovatriptan, naratriptan, rizatriptan, zolmitriptan*
‡*Early development stopped due to animal toxicity.*

Humans have at least seven 5-HT receptor subtypes (Tables 5.2, 5.3), and the triptan drugs are active at a number of these sub-types. As refinements of the triptan compounds are developed, the relevant receptor for anti-migraine activity will become clear.

How do the triptans work?

The possible modes of action of the triptans are illustrated in Figure 5.12. In essence, the triptans can act both in the peripheral arm of the trigemi-novascular system and on the central arm in the trigeminal nucleus. They can thus:

- constrict cranial vessels via activation of the 5HT$_{1B}$ vasoconstrictor receptor;
- inhibit peripheral trigeminal nerves by activation of the 5HT$_{1D}$ neuronal inhibitory receptor; and
- block pain signals in the trigeminal nucleus via activation of 5HT$_{1B/1D}$ receptors in the trigeminocervical complex.

It is not clear which, if any, of these mechanisms is dominant, although in terms of future development, it is crucial to know if a purely neuronal inhibitory approach is possible.

The future

Treatment responses to predictions made by pre-clinical studies of the various anti-migraine drugs in the experimental models help to define the pathophysiology of the disease. Some effort has been made to move away from drugs with a vas-cular action, which all of the 5-HT$_{1B/1D}$ agonist compounds possess, to more neuronally active compounds, such as CP122,288, substance P antagonists, and endothelin antagonists, although without success thus far. Ultimately, the question of whether non-vascularly active drugs can be developed must be answered in the quest for the ideal treatment.

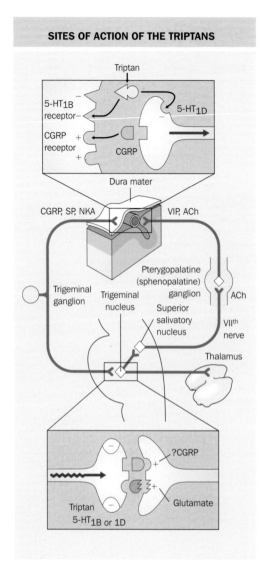

SITES OF ACTION OF THE TRIPTANS

Figure 5.12 *The possible sites of action of the triptans are illustrated. Triptans, $5HT_{1B/1D}$ agonists (see Table 5.3), have both peripheral and central sites of action. The peripheral sites are the cranial vessels via activation of the $5HT_{1B}$ vasoconstrictor receptor and the $5HT_{1D}$ neuronal inhibitory receptor. Also, $5HT_{1B/1D}$ receptors are found in the trigeminal nucleus and their activation inhibits pain signals as they enter the brainstem. (NMDA, N-methyl-D-aspartate; AMPA, α-amino-3-hydroxy-5-methylisoxazole-4-proprionic acid.)*

Studies suggest that trigeminal ganglia may preferentially contain 5-HT_{1D} receptors, and blood vessels preferentially contain 5-HT_{1B} receptors. Certainly, $5HT_{1B}$ receptors may be found in the coronary vessels, a target most clinicians would seek to avoid, and, therefore, non-vascular receptor targets would be attractive. For example, an exclusive 5-HT_{1D} agonist with only neuronal actions would be attractive, and although the first compound studied did not work. A specific 5-HT_{1F} is in clinical trials because it lacks vascular action, and preliminary results are encouraging. This research area is creating excitement.

Summary

- Understanding the basic anatomy and physiology of cranial circulation helps to assess and manage patients with headaches, particularly *neurovascular-type headaches*, such as migraine and cluster headache.
- Migraine should be viewed as an episodic syndrome of pain, probably involving intracranial structures and certainly associated with other neurological disturbances.
- The syndromic nature of migraine is its core characteristic, and the brain and connections that process and control head pain are responsible for that syndrome.
- The crucial sites in migraine are the aminergic nuclei, the role of which is to gate afferent nociceptive information, modulate CBF and blood–brain permeability, and control the signal-to-noise aspect of sensory inputs.
- The trigeminovascular system provides a therapeutic target for attack treatment because it arrests the final common pathway for expression of *neurovascular* head pain.
- The brain provides the essential key to migraine, its genesis, and ultimate understanding and control.

Further reading

Historical

Lashley KS. Patterns of cerebral integration indicated by the scotomas of migraine. *Arch Neurol Psychiatry* 1941; 46: 331–9.

Leao AAP. Spreading depression of activity in cerebral cortex. *J Neurophysiol* 1944; 7: 359–90.

Wolff HG. *Headache and Other Head Pain*. New York: Oxford University Press; 1963.

Modern

Beer M, Middlemiss D, Stanton J *et al*. *In vitro* pharmacological profile of the novel 5-HT$_{1D}$ receptor agonist MK-462. *Cephalalgia* 1995; 15 (Suppl. 14): 203.

Cutrer FM, Limmroth V, Woeber C, Yu X, Moskowitz MA. New targets for antimigraine drug development. In: Goadsby PJ, Silberstein SD (eds). *Headache*. Philadelphia: Butterworth–Heinemann, 1997: 59–120.

Ducros A, Joutel A, Vahedi K *et al*. Familial hemiplegic migraine: mapping of the second gene and evidence for a third locus. *Cephalalgia* 1997; 17: 232.

Edvinsson L, Goadsby PJ. Neuropeptides in headache. *Eur J Neurol* 1998: 5(4): 329–41.

Gardner K, Barmada M, Ptacek LJ, Hoffman EP. A new locus for hemiplegic maps to chromosome 1q31. *Neurology* 1997; 489: 1231–8.

Goadsby PJ. 5-HT$_{1B/1D}$ agonists in migraine: comparative pharmacology and its therapeutic implications. *CNS Drugs* 1998; 10: 271–86.

Goadsby PJ, Hoskin KL. The distribution of trigeminovascular afferents in the non-human primate brain *Macaca nemestrina*: a c-fos immunocytochemical study. *J. Anat* 1997; 190: 367–75.

Goadsby PJ, Silberstein SD. Headache. In: Asbury A, Marsden CD (eds). *Blue Books in Practical Neurology*, Vol. 17. New York: Butterworth–Heinemann, 1997.

Hoyer D, Clarke DE, Fozard JR *et al*. International Union of Pharmacology classification of receptors for 5-hydroxytryptamine (serotonin). *Pharmacol Rev* 1994; 46: 157–203.

Lance JW, Goadsby PJ. *Mechanism and Management of Headache*. London: Butterworth–Heinemann, 1998.

Lauritzen M. Pathophysiology of the migraine aura. The spreading depression theory. *Brain* 1994; 117: 199–210.

Ophoff RA, Terwindt GM, Vergouwe MN *et al*. Familial hemiplegic migraine and episodic ataxia type-2 are caused by mutations in the Ca^{2+} channel gene CACNLA4. *Cell* 1996; 87: 543–52.

Silberstein SD, Lipton RB, Goadsby PJ. *Headache in Clinical Practice*. Oxford: ISIS Medical Media, 1998.

Strassman AM, Raymond SA, Burstein R. Sensitization of meningeal sensory neurons and the origin of headaches. *Nature* 1996; 384: 560–3.

Weiller C, May A, Limmroth V *et al*. Brain stem activation in spontaneous human migraine attacks. *Nature Med* 1995; 1: 658–60.

Woods RP, Iacoboni M, Mazziotta JC. Bilateral spreading cerebral hypoperfusion during spontaneous migraine headache. *New Engl J Med* 1994; 331: 1689–92.

Primary headache disorders

6 Migraine: diagnosis and treatment

Introduction

Migraine is a primary episodic headache disorder characterized by various combinations of neurological, gastrointestinal, and autonomic changes. In the United States, more than 17% of women and 6% of men had at least one migraine attack in the past year. Many famous and creative individuals have suffered from migraine (Table 6.1). Migraine diagnosis is based on the retrospective reporting of headache characteristics and associated symptoms. Physical and neurological examination, as well as laboratory studies, are usually normal and serve to exclude other more ominous causes of headache (*see* Chapters 2 and 4). Formal diagnostic criteria for migraine and other headache disorders were published by the International Headache Society (IHS) in 1988. The IHS system recognizes seven subtypes of migraine with two major varieties: migraine without aura and migraine with aura (Table 6.2). In this chapter, the migraine attack and the acute and preventive treatment are described, based in part on the presence of coexistent or comorbid disease

Description of the migraine attack

The migraine attack can be divided into three phases (Figure 6.1):

- Phase I: premonitory phase – occurs hours or days before the headache;
- Phase II: main attack phase – consists of the headache, which may be seen in association with aura in about 15% of cases:
  - Phase IIA: aura phase: immediately precedes or occurs with the headache,
  - Phase IIB: headache phase;
- Phase III: headache resolution phase.

Most people experience more than one phase.

Phase I: premonitory phenomena

Premonitory phenomena may occur in up to 60% of migraineurs, although the precise incidence is unknown. These symptoms are seen with equal frequency in migraine with aura and migraine without aura. They often occur hours to days before headache onset. Usually, patients describe a characteristic change in mood or behaviour, which may include psychological, neurological, constitutional, or autonomic features (Table 6.3). Some people simply report a poorly characterized feeling that a migraine attack is coming.

● **Table 6.1** Some famous migraineurs

Julius Caesar	Thomas Jefferson	Ulysses S. Grant
Saint Paul	Friedrich Nietzsche	Peter Tchaikovsky
John Calvin	Immanuael Kant	Alfred Nobel
Queen Mary Tudor	Edgar Allan Poe	Leo Tolstoy
Blaise Pascal	Frédéric Chopin	Sigmund Freud
Carolus Linnaeus	Charles Darwin	Virginia Woolf
Lewis Carroll	Karl Marx	Princess Margaret

Adapted from Adler *et al.*, 1987

● **Table 6.2** IHS migraine classification

1	Migraine
1.1	Migraine without aura
1.2	Migraine with aura
1.2.1	Migraine with typical aura
1.2.2	Migraine with prolonged aura
1.2.3	Familial hemiplegic migraine
1.2.4	Basilar migraine
1.2.5	Migraine aura without headache
1.2.6	Migraine with acute onset aura
1.3	Ophthalmoplegic migraine
1.4	Retinal migraine
1.5	Childhood periodic syndromes that may be precursors to or associated with migraine
1.5.1	Benign paroxysmal vertigo of childhood
1.5.2	Alternating hemiplegia of childhood
1.6	Complications of migraine
1.6.1	Status migrainosus
1.6.2	Migrainous infarction
1.7	Migrainous disorder not fulfilling above criteria

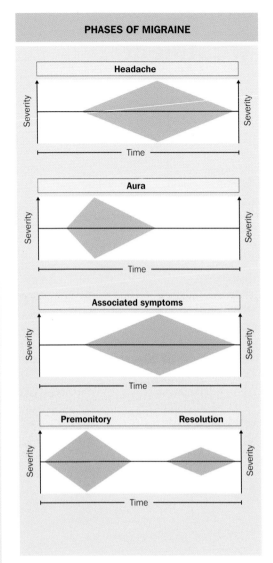

PHASES OF MIGRAINE

● **Table 6.3** Prodrome (premonitory phenomena)

Mental state	Neurological	General
Depressed	Photophobia	Stiff neck
Hyperactive	Difficulty concentrating	Food cravings
Euphoric	Phonophobia	Cold feeling
Talkative	Dysphasia	Anorexia
Irritable	Hyperosmia	Sluggish
Drowsy	Yawning	Diarrhoea or constipation
Restless		Thirst
		Urination
		Fluid retention

● **Table 6.4** Characteristics of the visual aura

Positive phenomena, negative phenomena, or both	Either may occur alone; positive phenomena often occur first and are followed by negative phenomena
Visual field	Scotoma often start centrally and migrate peripherally.
Shape	Fortification spectra are often 'C'-shaped; scotoma bean shaped
Motion	Objects may rotate, oscillate, or boil
Flicker	Rate of 10 cycles per second; may change during the course of the aura
Colour	Grey, red, green, gold, yellow, blue, or purple; often have no specific colour except excessively bright white
Clarity	May be blurry or fuzzy
Brightness	Often very bright
Expansion	Build-up occurs in both fortification spectra and scotoma
Migration	Spectra may 'march' from the central area to the periphery or sometimes vice versa

● **Figure 6.1** Phases of migraine attack.

While the prodromal features vary among individuals, they are often consistent within an individual. A diary may be helpful to show the relationship of these periodic events to migraine (Table 6.3 and Figure 6.3).

Phase II: main attack phase

Phase IIA: aura

The migraine aura is a complex of focal neurological symptoms (positive or negative phenomena) that precedes or accompanies an attack in about 15% of patients. Most aura symptoms develop over 5–20 minutes and usually last less than 60 minutes. The aura may have the following characteristics:

- visual, characterized by flashing jagged lights or visual loss (Table 6.4);
- sensory, with pins and needles on the face or involving the limbs;
- motor phenomena, such as weakness or incoordination;
- language problems, such as difficulty finding or using words; or
- brainstem disturbances, such as vertigo or double vision.

Headache usually occurs within 60 minutes of the end of the aura, but may not occur for several hours. Migraine auras may occur without headache,

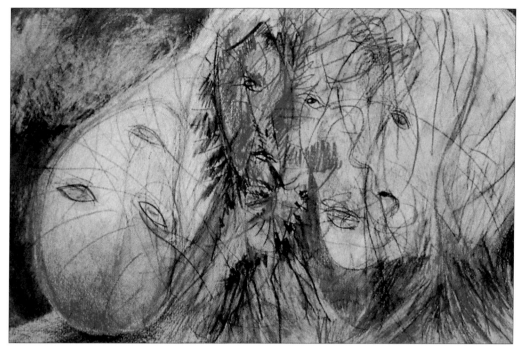

● **Figure 6.2** *'Mentally insufficient' by Angela Mark of Jamaica Plain, Massachusetts, USA. (© Sandoz Pharmaceuticals Corp.)*

EXAMPLE OF A MIGRAINE DIARY

	Date	Headache start time	Headache stop time	Severity (0–3 scale) 0 = none 1 = mild 2 = moderate 3 = severe	Associated symptoms (0–4 scale) 0 = none 1 = nausea 2 = vomiting 3 = photophobia 4 = phonophobia	Disability (0–3 scale) 0 = none 1 = mild 2 = moderate 3 = severe	Medications taken to relieve headache	Any known triggers
Sun								
Mon								
Tue								
Wed								
Thur								
Fri								
Sat								

● **Figure 6.3** *Example of a migraine diary.*

which raises the spectre of ocular pathology (retinal detachment) or seizures, among other causes. Most patients do not feel completely normal during the gap between the aura and the headache. Fears, somatic complaints, alterations in mood, disturbances of speech or thought, or detachment from the environment or from other people may occur. The headache may also begin before, or simultaneously with, the aura.

Patients can have more than one type of aura, with a progression from one symptom to another. Auras may occur repeatedly, many times a day, for weeks or months, but this presentation is rare and

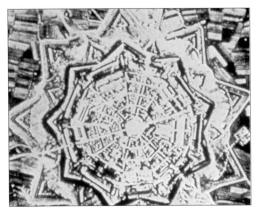

● **Figure 6.4** Migraine with aura (aerial view of the fortified, walled city of Palmanova, Italy.)

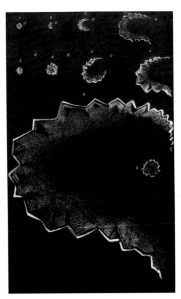

● **Figure 6.5** Scintillating scotomata. From Dr Hubert Airy's classic paper, 'On a distinct form of transient hemiopsia'.

requires referral to a specialist and careful investigation. Auras vary in complexity. Simple visual auras include scotomata (areas of visual loss), simple flashes (phosphenes), specks, or geometric forms. They may move across the visual field, sometimes crossing the midline, and are more likely to occur during than before the headache. Since they usually affect a visual field rather than one eye, they are believed to arise from the occipital cortex. More complicated auras include teichopsia (a Greek word meaning 'town wall' and 'vision') or fortification spectrum, the most characteristic visual aura of migraine (Figure 6.4). An arc of scintillating lights may start near a point of fixation and may form into a pattern like that of a herring-bone. The arc migrates across the visual field with a scintillating edge of often zig-zag, flashing, or occasionally coloured phenomena (Figure 6.5). Some characteristics of the aura, listed in Table 6.4, may occur simultaneously in both visual fields, but this is rare. The visions of Hildegard of Bingen, an 11th century mystic, have been attributed in part to her migrainous scintillating scotomas (Figure 6.6).

Visual distortions and hallucinations can occur and do so more commonly in children. They usually are followed by a headache and may be characterized by visual distortions and perversions of size and shape. Occasionally complex difficulties in the perception and use of the body (apraxia and agnosia), speech and language disturbances, states of double or multiple consciousness associated with deja vu or jamais vu, and elaborate, dreamy, nightmarish, trance-like, or delirious states may occur. When this happens, the differential diagnosis includes seizure, cerebrovascular disease, structural brain disease, and primary psychiatric disorders.

Paraesthesias (pins and needles), the second most common aura, typically start in the hand, migrate up the arm, and then jump to the face, lips, and tongue. The leg is occasionally involved. Paraesthesias may be followed by numbness and, in a few cases, loss of positional sense. Paraesthesias start or become bilateral in half of patients. Sensory auras rarely occur in isolation and usually follow a visual aura (Figure 6.7).

Motor symptoms can occur in up to 18% of patients with aura, most often in association with sensory symptoms; however, true weakness is rare and is always unilateral. Aphasic auras (speech abnormalities), including aphasia, have been reported in 17–20% of patients with aura. However, since patients are rarely examined during an aura, many of these reported cases may be dysarthria, not aphasia.

Phase IIB: pain phase

The typical migraine headache is unilateral, throbbing, moderate to severe in intensity, and aggravated by physical activity. Not all of these features are required to qualify as migraine; pain may be bilateral at onset (in 40% of cases) or start on one side and become generalized. The headache of migraine can occur at any time of the day or night, but it occurs most frequently on arising in the morning. The onset is usually gradual, the pain peaks, then subsides, and usually lasts between 4 and 72 hours in adults and 2 to 48 hours in children (Figure 6.8).

MIGRAINE AURA

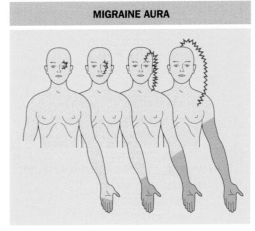

● **Figure 6.7** *Paraesthesias, the second most common migraine aura. (Adapted with permission from Spierings, 1996.)*

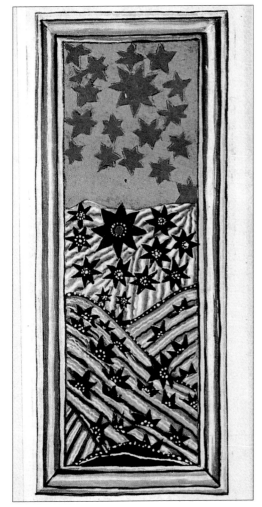

● **Figure 6.6** *'Vision of the fall of the angels' from a manuscript of Hildegard's Scivias, written in Bingen, AD 1180.*

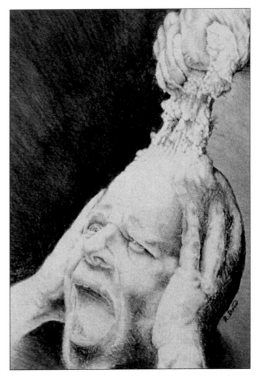

● **Figure 6.8** *'Gripping headache' by Richard Dorrow II of Athol, Massachusetts, USA. (© Sandoz Pharmaceuticals Corp.)*

The head pain varies greatly in intensity, although most people with migraine report pain ratings of 5 on a scale of 0 to 10. Patients describe their pain as throbbing in 85% of cases, although throbbing pain is often described in other types of headache. Physical activity or simple head movement commonly aggravates the pain.

Other features invariably accompany the pain of migraine. Anorexia is common, although food craving can also occur. Nausea occurs in up to 90% of patients, and vomiting with some attacks occurs in about one-third of migraineurs (Figure 6.9). Many patients experience sensory hyper-excitability manifested by photophobia, phono-phobia, and osmophobia. These patients often seek a dark, quiet room or take other steps to avoid light and sound (Figure 6.10). Other sys-temic symptoms, including blurry vision, nasal stuffiness, tenesmus, diarrhoea, abdominal cramps, polyuria (followed by decreased urinary output after the attack), pallor (or, less com-monly, redness) of the face, sensations of heat or cold, and sweating, may be noted during the headache phase. Impairment of concentration is common; less often there is memory impairment. Depression, fatigue, anxiety, nervousness, and irritability are common. Lightheadedness rather than true vertigo and a feeling of faintness may occur. The extremities tend to be cold and moist.

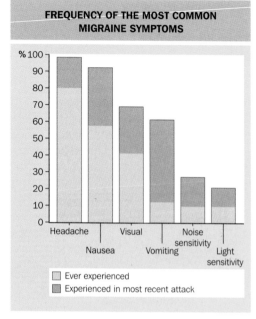

● **Figure 6.9** *Frequency of the most common migraine symptoms. (Adapted with permission from Silberstein, 1995.)*

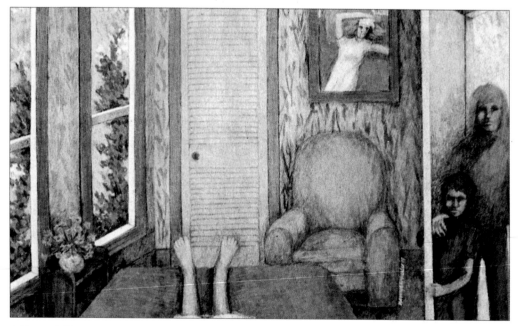

● **Figure 6.10** *'Serving time' by Nancy Ellen Wheeler of Scituate, Massachusetts, USA. (© Sandoz Pharmaceutical Corp.)*

Phase III: resolution phase

As the pain lessens, the patient may feel tired, washed out, irritable, and listless and may have impaired concentration, scalp tenderness, or mood changes. Some patients feel unusually refreshed or euphoric after an attack, while others experience depression and malaise.

Formal diagnostic criteria

The IHS classification of headache disorders was intended to improve clinical practice and research by clarifying previously vague definitions, so these diagnostic criteria are used in this discussion of migraine.

Migraine without aura (formerly common migraine)

Diagnosis of IHS migraine without aura (Table 6.5) requires:

- at least five lifetime attacks, with the features:
- attacks lasting 4–72 hours,
- two of these pain characteristics – unilateral location, pulsating quality, moderate-to-severe intensity, and aggravation by routine physical activity,
- at least one of nausea, vomiting, photophobia, or phonophobia;
- no evidence of organic disease.

binations of features are required, and exclusion, because alternative causes of headache must be systematically eliminated. Some patients who do not meet IHS criteria for migraine have recurrent primary headaches with migrainous features. These

● **Table 6.5** *Migraine without aura (previously used terms – common migraine, hemicrania simplex): diagnostic criteria*

A At least five attacks fulfilling B–D.

B Headache lasting 4–72 hours (untreated or unsuccessfully treated).

C Headache has at least two of the following characteristics:

  1 Unilateral location.

  2 Pulsating quality.

  3 Moderate or severe intensity (inhibits or prohibits daily activities).

  4 Aggravation by walking stairs or similar routine physical activity.

D During headache at least one of the following:

  1 Nausea and/or vomiting.

  2 Photophobia and phonophobia.

E At least one of the following:

  1 History, physical and neurological examinations do not suggest one of the disorders listed in IHS Groups 5–11.

  2 History and/or physical and/or neurological examinations do suggest such a disorder, but it is ruled out by appropriate investigations.

  3 Such a disorder is present, but migraine attacks do not occur for the first time in close temporal relation to the disorder.

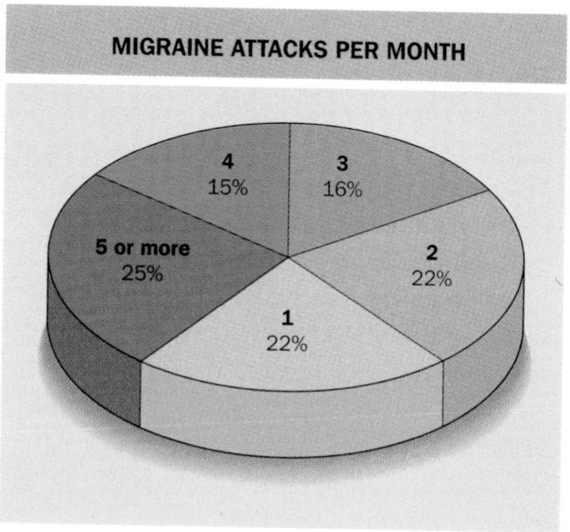

Migraine may last for several hours or all day, and when it persists for more than 3 days, it is called 'status migrainosus'. Migraine often begins in the morning, but it can begin at any time of the day or night. Frequency varies among individuals, from a few in a lifetime to several a week, with an average of 1–3 a month (Figure 6.11). The IHS qualification requirement of at least five lifetime attacks is imposed because headaches that simulate migraine may be caused by organic disease ranging from brain tumours to sinusitis to glaucoma. The IHS criteria require that secondary headache disorders be excluded, usually by history and physical examination, but on occasion through the judicious use of diagnostic tests. Migraine is thus a diagnosis of both inclusion, because specific com-

MIGRAINE ATTACKS PER MONTH

4 — 15%
3 — 16%
5 or more — 25%
2 — 22%
1 — 22%

● **Figure 6.11** *Frequency of migraine attacks experienced by migraineurs per month.*

patients may be missing just one IHS defining feature or may have other features, such as menstrual exacerbation or osmophobia, that strongly suggest migraine. Once secondary headache is excluded, we treat these patients as if they have migraine, but maintain a heightened index of diagnostic suspicion for other disorders.

Migraine with aura (classic migraine)

Diagnosis of migraine (Table 6.6) with aura requires:

- at least two lifetime attacks; and
- three of the following features:
  - one or more fully reversible aura symptoms,
  - aura developing over more than 4 minutes,
  - aura lasting less than 60 minutes,
  - headache following aura with a free interval of less than 60 minutes, and
  - no evidence of organic disease.

Migraine with aura can be subdivided into categories (*see* Table 6.2). The headache and associated symptoms of migraine with aura are similar to those of migraine without aura. Most migraineurs who have aura also have attacks without aura. In contrast to transient ischaemic attack and stroke, the aura of migraine often evolves gradually and consists of both positive (e.g. scintillations, tingling) and negative (e.g. scotoma, numbness) features. Focal symptoms and signs may persist beyond the headache phase.

Migraine variants

Migraine variants, while uncommon, are not rare.

Basilar migraine

Basilar migraine (Table 6.7) can present a confusing picture and is nothing more complex than an aura that affects the brainstem. It affects all age groups and both sexes, but usually begins in childhood and adolescence. The aura often lasts less than 1 hour, and is followed by a headache. The aura produces clinical features that reflect brainstem dysfunction, including ataxia, vertigo, tinnitus, diplopia, nausea, vomiting, nystagmus, dysarthria, bilateral paraesthesia, or a change in level of consciousness and cognition.

Confusional migraine

Confusional migraine is characterized by a typical aura, a headache (which may be insignificant), and confusion, which may precede the headache or follow it. The confusion is characterized by inattention, distractibility, and difficulty maintaining speech and other motor activities. This is nothing more than an aura that affects the centres controlling consciousness.

Hemiplegic migraine

Hemiplegic migraine can be sporadic or familial – both types typically begin in childhood and end in adulthood. The attacks are frequently

---

Table 6.6 *Migraine with aura (classic migraine): diagnostic criteria*

A At least two attacks fulfilling B.
B At least three of the following four characteristics:
1 One or more fully reversible aura symptoms indicating brain dysfunction.
2 At least one aura symptom develops gradually over more than 4 minutes or two or more symptoms occur in succession.
3 No single aura symptom lasts more than 60 minutes.
4 Headache follows aura with a free interval of less than 60 minutes (it may also begin before or simultaneously with the aura).
C History, physical examination, and, where appropriate, diagnostic tests exclude a secondary cause.

Table 6.7 *Basilar migraine: diagnostic criteria*

Description: Migraine with aura symptoms clearly originating from the brainstem or from both occipital lobes
A Fulfils criteria for migraine with aura (Table 6.6)
B Two or more aura symptoms of the following types:
Visual symptoms in both the temporal and nasal fields of both eyes
Dysarthria
Vertigo
Tinnitus
Decreased hearing
Double vision
Ataxia
Bilateral paraesthesias
Bilateral pareses
Decreased level of consciousness

● **Table 6.8** *Familial hemiplegic migraine: diagnostic criteria*

Description:
Migraine with aura including hemiparesis and where at least one first-degree relative has identical attacks.

A Fulfils criteria for migraine with aura (Table 6.6)

B The aura includes some degree of hemiparesis and may be prolonged.

C At least one first-degree relative has identical attacks.

● **Table 6.9** *Comparison of familial hemiplegic migraine, cerebral autosomal dominant arteriopathy with subcortical infarcts and leukoencephalopathy and migraine with white matter abnormalities*

	FHM	CADASIL	Migraine with white matter abnormalities
Genetics	AD	AD	AD
Chromosomal locus	19*, ?	19	19 (?)
MRI	WNL	ABN	ABN
Migraine	Yes	Yes	Yes
Migraine with aura and hemiparesis	Yes	Yes	Yes
Stroke	No	Yes	No
Dementia	No	Yes	No

* When associated with cerebellar abnormalities.

precipitated by minor head injury. Changes in consciousness that range from confusion to coma are a feature of hemiplegic migraine, especially in childhood. The hemiplegia may be part of the aura or it may last for days or weeks, and headache may precede the hemiparesis or it may be absent. The onset of hemiparesis may be abrupt and simulate a stroke or transient ischaemic attack. It may be difficult to differentiate migraine from vascular disease with the first attack. A full neurological evaluation is needed to seek causes of stroke in young people. Estimates of the frequency of hemiplegic migraine vary from 4–30% of cases of migraine. The differential diagnosis includes stroke, homocystinuria, focal seizures, and MELAS syndrome (migraine, epilepsy, lactic acidosis, and stroke), which is a mitochondrial disorder.

Familial hemiplegic migraine

Familial hemiplegic migraine (FHM; Table 6.8) has an autosomal dominant mode of inheritance, and results from more than one genetic abnormality. The gene has been localized in some families and the defect found to result from an abnormality in a brain-specific P/Q voltage-gated calcium-channel subunit (*see* Chapter 5).

CADASIL

Cerebral autosomal dominant arteriopathy with subcortical infarcts and leukoencephalopathy (CADASIL) is a rare inherited arterial disease of the brain; it was recently mapped (in several unrelated families) to a gene that codes for a notch protein on chromosome 19 (Table 6.9). The complete CADASIL syndrome consists of recurrent strokes that start in mid-adult life and often lead to dementia, residual motor disability, and pseudobulbar palsy. The definition of CADASIL is migraine with aura and some hemiparesis, when the patient has at least one first-degree relative with identical attacks. It can be diagnosed by characteristic MRI abnormalities (Figure 6.12)

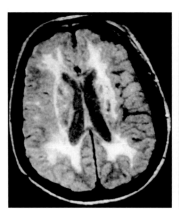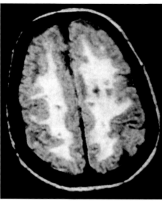

● **Figure 6.12** *MRI CADASIL. Brain MRI showing axial proton density sections at the level of the bodies of the lateral ventricles and centrum, which show confluent, severe, high-signal leukoencephalopathy, with discrete punctate low-signal lesions indicating cystic or necrotic lesions. (Reproduced with permission from Hutchinson et al., 1995.)*

in a genetically at-risk family member who has a pattern of autosomal dominant inheritance. The main clinical representation of CADASIL is recurrent subcortical events, either transient or (more often) permanent.

Migraine with white matter abnormalities

Physicians are frequently confronted with MRI reports of white matter abnormalities (WMA) in migraine patients, which can cause concern to both the patient and the doctor. These are not uncommon in migraine, particularly migraine with aura, but the exact cause is not known. One theory is that WMA and migraine with aura are caused by the same underlying vascular disorder that is present in mitochondrial diseases or the antiphospholipid antibody syndrome. Another theory is that a mutation near the CADASIL locus is a new cause of migraine associated with WMA, as seen on MRI (Table 6.9). If the patient has typical migraine that meets IHS criteria and no other neurological signs and symptoms, further investigation is probably not needed. However, if the neurological examination is abnormal and the patient has hemiplegic migraine, basilar migraine, migraine with a prolonged aura, or a family history of any of these disorders, a neurological consultation may be indicated.

Aura without headache

Periodic neurological dysfunction, which may be part of the migraine aura, can occur in isolation without the headache. These phenomena (scintillating scotomata and/or recurrent sensory, motor, and mental phenomena) often occur in patients who usually also have headaches associated with their auras. Fisher described late-life migrainous accompaniments (occurring in patients older than 40 years of age), which are transient neurological phenomena not associated with headache (Table 6.10). Most patients with late-life migraine accompaniments are men, and most have had a history of migraine. They had one or more attacks of episodic neurological dysfunction with variable recurrence. Fisher felt that scintillating scotoma was diagnostic of migraine even when it occurred in isolation, whereas other episodic neurological symptoms (paraesthesias, aphasia, and sensory and motor symptoms) needed more careful evaluation (Table 6.11).

● **Table 6.10** *Main criteria for the diagnosis of late-life migrainous accompaniments (Fisher)*

- Scintillations (or other visual display), paraesthesias, aphasia, dysarthria and paralysis.
- Build-up of scintillations; not seen in cerebrovascular disease.
- 'March' of paraesthesias; not seen in cerebrovascular disease.
- Progression from one accompaniment to another, often with a delay.
- Two or more similar attacks; helps exclude embolism.
- Headache occurs in 50% of attacks.
- Episodes last 15–25 minutes.
- Characteristic mid-life 'flurry' of attacks.
- Generally benign course.
- Normal angiography: excludes thrombosis.
- Rule out: cerebral thrombosis, embolism and dissection, epilepsy, thrombocythemia, polycythemia, and thrombotic thrombocytopenia.

(Adapted from Fisher CM)

● **Table 6.11** *Migrainous accompaniments*

Visual-scintillating scotoma	Hemiplegia
Ophthalmoplegia	Cyclical vomiting
Paraesthesias	Brainstem symptoms
Oculosympathetic palsy	Seizures
Aphasia	Blindness
Mydriasis	Diplopia
Dysarthria	Blurring of vision
Confusion-stupor	Deafness
Dizziness	Hemianopia
Recurrence of old stroke deficit	

Treatment

Effective migraine treatment includes the following:

- making an accurate diagnosis;
- explaining the condition to the patient (allaying fears, displaying interest, explaining the difference between curing and long-term control of migraine and the role of the patient in treatment);
- developing a treatment plan that considers diagnosis, symptoms, comorbid conditions (comorbid conditions may include stroke, epilepsy, mitral valve prolapse, Raynaud's syndrome, and

● **Table 6.12** *Migraine comorbid disease*

Cardiovascular	Neurological	Gastrointestinal tract	Psychiatric	Other
Hyper- or hypotension	Epilepsy	Functional bowel disorders	Depression	Asthma
Raynaud's phenomenon	Positional vertigo		Mania	Allergies
Mitral valve prolapse			Panic disorder	
Angina/myocardial infarction			Anxiety disorder	
Stroke				

psychological disorders, such as depression, mania, anxiety and panic; Table 6.12); and

- setting priorities to deal with the symptoms most disturbing to the patient.

It is important to establish a specific diagnosis prior to treatment. A migraine-specific medication may be useless or even dangerous if used to treat a condition that looks like, but is not, migraine. For example, a patient with acute symptomatic headache caused by a stroke or subarachnoid haemorrhage may respond to a triptan with a worsened neurological deficit. For that reason, treatment should not be used as a diagnostic test.

A headache calendar (diary), in which patients record the duration and severity of their headaches as well as their response to treatment, is a very useful tool. Non-pharmacological treatment, such as relaxation, biofeedback, and the behavioural interventions outlined in Table 6.13, are important, particularly for children, pregnant women, and patients in whom stress is a trigger.

Although behavioural interventions are important, drugs are the mainstay of treatment for most patients (Table 6.14). Pharmacological treatment may be acute (abortive) or preventive (prophylactic), and patients who experience frequent severe headaches often require both approaches.

The physician should consider the following points about acute treatment:

- acute medications include analgesics, antiemetics, anxiolytics, non-steroidal anti-inflammatory drugs (NSAIDs), ergots, corticosteroids, major tranquillizers, opioids, and triptans (selective 5-hydroxytryptamine [5-HT$_1$] agonists);

- acute medications can be non-specific or specific (Table 6.15): non-specific medications work for headache and other pain, while specific medications work only for head pain;
- acute (abortive) headache medication is intended to relieve the pain and disability of an acute attack and stop its progression;
- patients who take preventive medication can also take acute medication during a headache; and
- to avoid rebound headache, patients should limit acute medication to only 2–3 days a week.

The following points refer to preventive therapy:

- preventive medications include beta-blockers, calcium-channel blockers, antidepressants, serotonin antagonists, anticonvulsants, and NSAIDs; and
- preventive therapy is given even in the absence of headache to reduce the frequency and perhaps the severity of anticipated attacks.

● **Table 6.13** *Behavioural modifications*

May help	Less likely to help
Regular sleep	Avoid milk products
Regular exercise	Avoid citrus products
Regular meals	
Avoid chocolate	
Avoid tyramine-containing food	
Avoid monosodium glutamate	
Avoid alcoholic beverages	
Limit caffeine	
Limit medications	
Biofeedback or stress management	

● **Table 6.14** Acute medications: efficacy, side effects, relative contraindications and indications

Drug	Efficacy*	Side effect*	Comorbid	
			Relative contraindications	Relative indications
Acetaminophen (paracetamol)	1+	1+	Liver disease	Pregnancy
Aspirin	1+	1+	Kidney disease, ulcer disease, PUD, gastritis (age <15 years)	CAD, TIA
Butalbital, caffeine and analgesics	2+	2+	Use of other sedative; history of medication overuse	
Caffeine adjuvant	2+	1+	Sensitivity to caffeine	
Isometheptene	2+	1+	Uncontrolled hypertension, CAD, PVD	
Opioids	3+	3+	Drug or substance abuse	Pregnancy; rescue medication
NSAIDs	2+	1+	Kidney disease, PUD, gastritis	
Dihydroergotamine				
Injections	4+	2+	CAD, PVD, uncontrolled hypertension prominent nausea or vomiting	Orthostatic hypotension
Intranasal	3+	1+		
Ergotamine				
Tablets	2+	2+	Prominent nausea or vomiting, CAD, PVD, uncontrolled hypertension	
Suppositories	3+	3+		
Sumatriptan				
SC Injection	4+	1+	CAD, PVD, uncontrolled hypertension	Prominent nausea or vomiting
Intranasal	3+	1+	CAD, PVD, uncontrolled hypertension	Prominent nausea or vomiting
Tablets	3+	1+	CAD, PVD, uncontrolled hypertension	Prominent nausea
Zolmitriptan				
Tablets	3+	1+	CAD, PVD, uncontrolled hypertension	Prominent nausea
Eletriptan				
Tablets	3+	1+	CAD, PVD, uncontrolled hypertension	Prominent nausea
Naratriptan				
Tablets	2+	1+	CAD, PVD, uncontrolled hypertension	Prominent nausea
Rizatriptan				
Tablets	3+	1+	CAD, PVD, uncontrolled hypertension	Prominent nausea

*Ratings are on a scale from 1+ (lowest) to 4+ (highest) based on response rates and consistency of response in double-blind placebo-controlled trials and our clinical experience.
PUD = peptic ulcer disease; PVD = peripheral vascular disease; CAD = coronary artery disease;
TIA = transient ischaemic attack; NSAIDs = non-steroidal anti-inflammatory drugs; SC = subcutaneous

● **Table 6.15** Migraine treatment

Acute (symptomatic)	Specific	For migraine only
	Non-specific	For any pain disorder or associated symptoms
Preventive (prophylactic)	Episodic	Immediately prior to triggering event
	Subacute	For limited time
	Chronic	Continuous

Optimizing therapy requires knowing about alternative treatments and understanding the patient's preferences. For example, some patients want to minimize their attack frequency and are willing to accept significant drug side effects to achieve this goal. Some patients are eager to try new therapies, while others are afraid to change an established regimen, even one with limited benefits. Some patients accept parenteral routes of administration readily, while others reject the idea of injections or suppositories.

Acute treatment

Many acute treatments are available for migraine (Figure 6.13). The choice depends on the severity and frequency of the headaches, the pattern

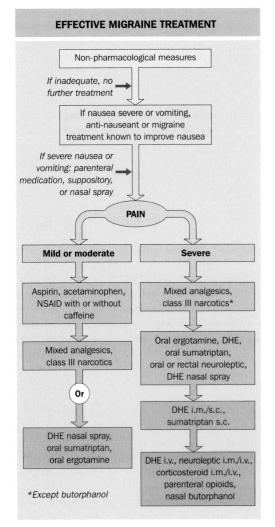

EFFECTIVE MIGRAINE TREATMENT

● **Figure 6.13** *Effective migraine treatment begins with making an accurate diagnosis. (DHE = dihydroergotamine.)*

ERGOTAMINE AND DIHYDROERGOTAMINE

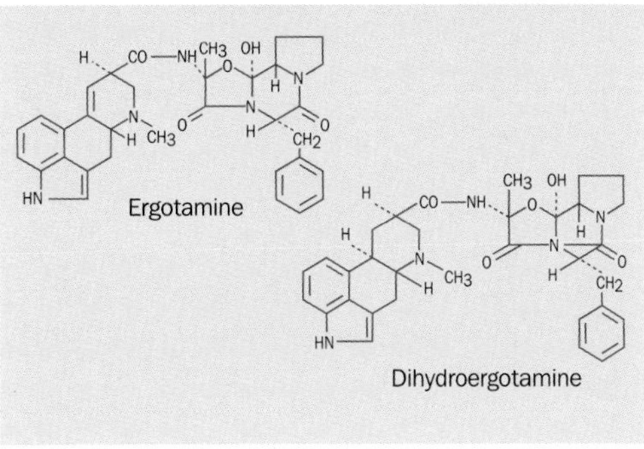

● **Figure 6.14** *Molecular structure of ergotamine and dihydroergotamine.*

headache. We also use the combination of paracetamol, isometheptene (a sympathomimetic), and dichloralphenazone (a chloral hydrate derivative). For patients with nausea or lack of effect with analgesics, we add antiemetics. When available, we prefer domperidone because it causes few central nervous system (CNS) problems. In the United States, domperidone is not available, and we use metoclopramide as a back-up. We often try naproxen sodium first, but we use other NSAIDs, often in combination with an antiemetic. Indomethacin, which is available as a 50 mg rectal suppository, and intramuscular ketorolac are useful for patients with severe nausea and vomiting.

Ergotamine and dihydroergotamine

We sometimes use ergotamine (Figure 6.14) and frequently use its derivative, dihydroergotamine (DHE), to treat moderate-to-severe migraine if analgesics do not provide satisfactory headache relief or if they produce significant side effects. Since rectal absorption is more reliable than oral, we prefer the suppository form of ergotamine. Patients who cannot tolerate ergotamine because of nausea are pretreated with an antiemetic. This problem can often be overcome by starting with one-half or one-third of the usual 2 mg ergotamine suppository; we routinely use this approach.

The derivative DHE has fewer side effects than ergotamine and can be administered intranasally (i.n.), intramuscularly (i.m.), subcutaneously (s.c.), or intravenously (i.v.); DHE is given in doses of up to 1 mg i.m. or i.v. per treatment with a maximum of 3 mg/day, or 2 mg i.n. per treatment with a

of the associated symptoms, the presence of comorbid illnesses, and the patient's treatment response profile (Table 6.14).

Simple and combination analgesics, and NSAIDs

We often begin with simple analgesics for patients with mild-to-moderate headaches. Many individuals find headache relief with a simple analgesic, such as aspirin or paracetamol (acetaminophen), either alone or in combination with caffeine. Butalbital is another effective analgesic adjuvant, but it is not available outside the United States. Caution is necessary with both caffeine and barbiturate combinations because of the risk of rebound maximum of 4 mg/day. We limit monthly use to 18 ampoules or 12 events, but when such levels of use are approached additional prophylactic medication is usually indicated. The headache recurrence rate with DHE is low (less than 20%), and it is less likely than ergotamine to exacerbate nausea or produce rebound headache.

Ergotamine and DHE should be avoided in women who are attempting to become pregnant and in patients with uncontrolled hypertension, sepsis, renal or hepatic failure, and coronary, cerebral, or peripheral vascular disease. While nausea is a common side effect of ergotamine, it is less common with DHE (unless it is given intravenously). Other side effects include dizziness, paraesthesias, abdominal cramps, and chest tightness; rare idiosyncratic arterial and coronary vasospasm can occur. We recommend an electrocardiogram before the first dose of ergotamine or DHE if there are any cardiac risk factors (including age of more than 40 years).

Selective 5-HT$_1$ agonists (triptans)

Sumatriptan

Sumatriptan (Figure 6.15) has been available as a subcutaneous injection and oral tablet since the early 1990s and, more recently, as a nasal spray. Its importance as a breakthrough therapy is demonstrated by the large number of pharmacologically related agents that followed it. Sumatriptan is the most extensively studied agent in the history of this disorder, with over 27,000 patients and over 140,000 attacks treated in the context of clinical trials up to May 1997.

Sumatriptan relieves headache pain, nausea, photophobia, and phonophobia, and restores the patient's ability to function normally. We often prescribe sumatriptan (or another triptan) at the

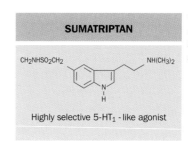

SUMATRIPTAN

CH$_2$NHSO$_2$CH$_2$ ... NH(CH$_3$)$_2$

Highly selective 5-HT$_1$ - like agonist

● *Figure 6.15* Molecular structure of sumatriptan.

initial consultation as a first-line drug for severe attacks and as an escape medication for less severe attacks that do not adequately respond to simple or combination analgesics. We prefer subcutaneous injection or nasal spray for patients who need rapid relief or who have severe nausea or vomiting. Oral sumatriptan is used for gradual-onset headache when rapid pain relief is not required. Although 80% of patients obtain pain relief from an initial subcutaneous dose of sumatriptan, headache recurs in about one-third of patients within a day. Recurrences respond well to a second dose of sumatriptan and sometimes to simple and combination analgesics.

Sumatriptan (and all the triptans) should not be used for patients who have clinical ischaemic heart disease, Prinzmetal's angina, uncontrolled hypertension, or strictly vertebrobasilar migraine or who are at high risk for these conditions. Sumatriptan's common side effects include pain at the injection site, tingling, flushing, burning, and warm or hot sensations. Dizziness, heaviness, neck pain, and dysphoria can also occur. These side effects generally abate within 45 minutes. Sumatriptan causes non-cardiac chest pressure in approximately 4% of patients. Before using any of the triptans, we obtain an electrocardiogram for patients over 40 years of age and for those who have risk factors for heart disease. We often

● **Table 6.16** Selective serotonin agonists

Action	Sumatriptan	Rizatriptan	Zolmitriptan	Naratriptan	Eletriptan
5-HT$_{1B/1D}$ affinity	✔	✔	✔	✔	✔
Cranial vasoconstrictor	✔	✔	✔	✔	✔
Coronary vasoconstrictor	✔	✔	✔	✔	✔
Inhibitor NI	✔	✔	✔	✔	✔
CNS penetration	–	✔	✔	✔	✔

NI = neurogenic inflammation

give the first triptan dose in the office at a time when the patient does not have a headache.

Second-generation triptans

Acute migraine treatment advanced significantly with the introduction of sumatriptan, the first specific $5\text{-HT}_{1B/1D}$ agonist (Table 6.16); however, there is still room for improvement. After oral administration of the drug, approximately half of patients do not respond at 2 hours, and about three-quarters have at least some residual headache pain. About one-third of patients using the oral formulation experience a headache recurrence within a day. A number of new $5\text{-HT}_{1B/1D}$ agonists (triptans), whose mechanism of action is similar to that of sumatriptan, but whose pharmacokinetics differ, have been developed. At least three are now in clinical use in North America and Europe. These may produce better migraine response rates and lower recurrence, and they may be better tolerated (Table 6.17).

Each compound has been shown in experimental settings to constrict extracerebral intracranial vessels, inhibit activity in peripheral trigeminal neurons, and, since each can penetrate the CNS to some extent, block transmission in the trigeminal nucleus. Also, each compound can constrict the human coronary artery, albeit to a very modest degree. The pharmacological characteristics of the triptans and their comparable efficacy are given in Tables 6.18 and 6.19.

Oral eletriptan is rapidly absorbed, with high bioavailability (50%) and a long half-life (4–5 h). In a dose-ranging, comparative trial, 2-hour responses were 54% at 20 mg, 65% at 40 mg and 77% at 80 mg with excellent therapeutic gains. In this study, recurrence rates were about one-third, similar to those of sumatriptan. The 80 mg dose was superior to 100 mg of sumatriptan. Response rates at 1 hour were 41% for eletriptan 80 mg, 38% for eletriptan 40 mg, 24% eletriptan 20 mg, 20% for

● **Table 6.17** Potential areas of improvement for oral sumatriptan

Area for clinical improvement	Hypothesized pharmacological property
Greater efficacy	CNS penetration
	Shorter T_{max}
Faster onset	Shorter T_{max}
Low recurrence rate	Longer half-life
	CNS penetration
Greater consistency	Improved bioavailability
Not metabolized by monoamine oxidase inhibitors	Fewer interactions
Neural selectivity (5-HT$_{1D}$)	Greater safety

● **Table 6.18** Pharmacological characteristics of selected triptans

Parameter	Sumatriptan	Zolmitriptan	Naratriptan	Rizatriptan	Eletriptan
Tmax (h)	2	2.5	2–3	1	1.5
Half-life (h)	2	3	6	2–3	4–5
Bioavailability (%)	14	40	60–70	40–45	50
Lipophilicity (log $D_{pH7.4}$)	–1.3	–0.7	0.2	0.7	+0.5

● **Table 6.19** Headache response and therapeutic gain for selected triptans at 2 hours

Triptan	Headache response at 2 h		Therapeutic gain* for response at 2 h	
	Average (%)	Range (%)	Average (%)	Range (%)
Sumatriptan (50 mg)	56	51–61	33	29–36
Zolmitriptan (2.5 mg)	64	59–69	34	27–41
Naratriptan (2.5 mg)	48	45–51	21	18–24
Rizatriptan (10 mg)	73	69–73	34	30–38
Eletriptan (80 mg)	72	67–77	45	36–53

*Therapeutic gain is the difference between the response to active drug and the response to placebo. It can be used to compare drugs tested in different clinical trials and is presented here with 95% confidence intervals based on published and abstracted studies.

sumatriptan 100 mg, and 12% for placebo. In this study, the most common treatment related adverse events were asthenia, paresthesia, nausea, and dizziness, and were dose related, mild and transient in nature. Eletriptan's phase III results are now becoming publicly available and along with direct comparator studies will help to establish its place in therapy. In a recently reported phase III study, 2-hour response rates of eletriptan 80 mg (67%) and 40 mg (64%) were statistically superior to sumatriptan 100 mg (53%), sumatriptan 50 mg (50%), and placebo (31%). Headache recurrence rates were 16% and 19% for the 80 and 40 mg doses respectively, compared to sumatriptan 100 mg (27), sumatriptan 50 mg (26%), and placebo (25%).

Oral naratriptan differs from sumatriptan primarily in its longer half-life, longer time to peak plasma concentration (T_{max}), higher oral bioavailability (70%), and lipophilicity. Studies of over 4000 patients indicate that the drug has a well-defined dose–response relationship for headache relief, with a mean response of 48% at 2 hours after administration, but therapeutic gains are comparatively modest (21%). In a direct comparative cross-over study with sumatriptan in patients prone to headache recurrence, about one-third fewer experienced recurrence when they used naratriptan compared with sumatriptan. The studies showed excellent tolerability for the 2.5 mg dose of naratriptan, with an adverse-event rate close to that of placebo.

Rizatriptan has high oral bioavailability, at 45% for the 10 mg dose, and rapid oral absorption. When directly compared with sumatriptan 100 mg, rizatriptan 10 mg had a cumulative benefit in terms of about 20% of patients achieving headache response in the first 2 hours and a cumulative advantage of about 15% when compared with sumatriptan 50 mg. Rizatriptan has high consistency from attack to attack in formal blinded consistency studies and a useful wafer (Melt®) formulation that many patients, particularly those with nausea as a prominent feature, find convenient as it dissolves on the tongue and requires no water. Rizatriptan has a significant interaction with propranolol, which requires that the dose be halved to 5 mg, and is contraindicated with monoamine oxidase inhibitors (MAOIs) because of its route of metabolism.

Zolmitriptan was the second selective 5-HT$_{1B/1D}$ agent marketed in the United States. It has high oral bioavailability (40%), a T_{max} of about 2.5 h, and metabolism by the cytochrome P450 system into an active metabolite, which is degraded by MAO-A. Therefore, patients taking MAOIs are limited to a total zolmitriptan dose of 5 mg/day. In studies, zolmitriptan demonstrated a headache response of 64%, with a therapeutic gain of 34%, for the 2.5 mg dose and headache response of 65%, with a 37% therapeutic gain, for the 5 mg dose. The recommended starting dose of 2.5 mg provides the best balance of benefit and side effects, although some patients may benefit from the higher 5 mg dose. In all studies, zolmitriptan reduced the incidence of photophobia, phonophobia, and nausea compared with placebo. In formal comparisons with sumatriptan 100 mg, zolmitriptan 5 mg was no different, and in a recent comparison with zolmitriptan 2.5 mg no clinically relevant differences were seen. The most frequently reported adverse events include asthenia, nausea, somnolence, dizziness, and paraesthesias. Table 6.20 indicates which triptan to choose in given situations.

Opioids

We use opioids but only when non-opioid medications do not provide adequate pain relief, if triptans or ergots are contraindicated, and as a back-up or rescue medication if the first treatment fails. We often start with codeine in combination with simple analgesics and sometimes butalbital or caffeine in the United States. In restrictive circumstances under which consumption can be monitored, we also sometimes use more potent opioid analgesics, such as propoxyphene, butorphanol, pethidine (meperidine), morphine, hydromorphone, and oxycodone, alone or in combination with simple analgesics. The use of such compounds can be difficult and is probably best carried out with the advice and regular supervision of a neurologist or headache specialist. We limit the amount of drug given, do not give refills, and insist on being the only source of prescription for the patient. Since medication overuse and rebound headache pose a threat with opioid use, these agents are most appropriate for patients whose severe headaches are relatively infrequent. Opiates that are mixed agonist–antagonists, such as butorphanol, have a lower drug abuse potential, although it is not clear if these agents offer any

● **Table 6.20** *Clinical stratification of acute specific migraine treatments*

Clinical situation	Treatment options
Failed analgesics and/or NSAIDs	*First tier*
	Sumatriptan 50 mg per os (p.o.)
	Rizatriptan 10 mg p.o.
	Zolmitriptan 2.5 mg p.o.
	Eletriptan 40 mg p.o.
	Dihydroergotamine 2 mg nasal spray
	Second tier
	Naratriptan 2.5 mg
	Ergotamine 1 mg p.o. or per rectum (p.r.; if headache infrequent)
Early nausea or problem taking tablets	Sumatriptan 20 mg nasal spray
	Sumatriptan 6 mg s.c.
	Rizatriptan 10 mg Melt® wafer
	Dihydroergotamine 2 mg nasal spray
	Dihydroergotamine 1 mg i.m., s.c.
Headache recurrence or long-lasting headache	Ergotamine (perhaps most effective p.r.)
	Naratriptan 2.5 mg p.o.
	Eletriptan 40 mg p.o.
	Dihydroergotamine 2 mg nasal spray
	Dihydroergotamine 1 mg i.m., s.c.
Tolerating triptans poorly	Naratriptan 2.5 mg
	Dihydroergotamine 2 mg nasal spray
Early vomiting	Sumatriptan 25 mg p.r. (available in Europe)
	Sumatriptan 6 mg s.c.
	Dihydroergotamine 2 mg nasal spray
	Dihydroergotamine 1 mg i.m., s.c.
Very rapidly developing symptoms	Sumatriptan 6 mg s.c.
	Dihydroergotamine 1 mg i.m., s.c.

● **Table 6.21** *Oral doses of opioid analgesics that achieve the same pain relief as 10 mg parenteral morphine for severe pain*

Drug		Oral dose (mg)	Oral-to-parenteral dose ratio	Parenteral dose (mg)
Morphine	Single dose	60	6:1	10
	Repeated dose	30	3:1	10
Hydromorphone		7.5	5:1	1.5
Methadone		2:0	2:1	
Levorphanol		4	2:1	
Pethidine (meperidine)		300	4:1	75
Codeine		200	1:5:1	130

of the night with a headache. Sedation, which is sometimes an undesirable side effect, may help the patient go back to sleep and awaken headache-free in the morning.

Adjunctive treatment

Nausea and vomiting can be as disabling as the headache itself. Gastric stasis and delayed gastric emptying decrease the effectiveness of oral medication. We use metoclopramide (10 mg in the United States) or domperidone (10 mg) as an antiemetic and a prokinetic to enhance the absorption of oral medications. Promethazine and ondansetron (a selective $5\text{-}HT_3$-receptor antagonist) i.v. (0.15 mg/kg diluted in 50 ml of 5% dextrose or normal saline) or orally (8 mg tablet) can be used by patients who cannot tolerate metoclopramide because of side effects. For nausea, vomiting, and pain, we use neuroleptics (chlorpromazine and prochlorperazine) intravenously, intramuscularly, and by suppository. Prochlorperazine suppositories (25 mg) are used as a primary treatment for headache and nausea as well as a rescue medication.

Preventive treatment

Preventive medications are given on a daily basis, whether or not headache is present, to reduce the frequency or severity of attacks. Preventive medication is usually taken daily for months or years, and treatment can be episodic, subacute (short-term), or chronic. Given the natural variation in migraine, it is wise to review all preventatives from time to time, probably every 6 months, but cer-

protection from rebound headache. Transnasal butorphanol tartrate (1 mg followed by 1 mg 1 hour later) is an effective acute outpatient treatment that rapidly relieves the pain of migraine and circumvents problems with oral absorption. Opiates should not be used on more than 2 days a week (Table 6.21).

In specific groups of patients, such as women with intractable menstrual migraine, we use narcotics on a more regular basis. These drugs are also especially helpful to patients who either do not respond to simple analgesics or who cannot take ergots or sumatriptan. Pregnant women can use codeine or pethidine with caution and in consultation with their obstetrician. Opioids are also useful for patients who awaken in the middle tainly yearly. Episodic preventive treatment is used when the headache trigger is known, such as exercise or sexual activity. Patients are instructed to pre-treat prior to the exposure or activity. For example, single doses of indomethacin can be used to prevent exercise-induced migraine. Subacute (short-term) preventive treatments are used in patients with a time-limited exposure to a trigger, such as menstruation. These patients can be treated with daily medication. For example, NSAIDs can be used perimenstrually before and during the exposure. Preventive medication can also be taken on a regular basis (chronic treatment) to decrease the frequency of migraine attacks.

Chronic preventive treatment should be considered in the following circumstances:

- when there is significant headache-related disability (e.g. two or more attacks a month that produce disability lasting 3 days or more);
- when acute medications are contraindicated, produce intolerable side effects, or are ineffective;
- when acute medications are being overused; or
- in special circumstances, such as hemiplegic migraine or rare headache attacks that produce profound disruption or risk of permanent neurological injury.

Preventive treatment should be avoided in the pregnant patient if possible. She must have severe disabling attacks accompanied by nausea, vomiting, and possibly dehydration before chronic preventive treatment is recommended, since the benefit must clearly outweigh the risks of treatment. Specialist consultation with the patient's obstetrician is advisable in this setting.

The major medication groups for preventive migraine treatment include beta-adrenergic blockers, antidepressants, calcium channel antagonists, serotonin antagonists, anticonvulsants, NSAIDs, and other agents. If preventive medication is indicated, the agent should be chosen from one of the major categories based on the side-effect profiles of the drugs and coexistent and comorbid conditions of the patient (Table 6.22).

Preventive medications should be started at a low dose and increased slowly until therapeutic effects develop or the ceiling dose for the agent is reached. Migraineurs frequently require a lower dose of a preventive medication than is needed for other indications. While doses of 75–200 mg/day of tricyclic antidepressants (TCAs), such as amitriptyline, are used to treat depression, 10–75 mg/day may be sufficient for migraine. In addition, migraineurs may be more sensitive to the side effects of medication. While a starting dose of 25–50 mg/day of amitriptyline is commonly used for patients with depression, that dose may produce intolerable side effects in migraineurs. Similarly, sodium valproate (divalproex sodium) is often effective at a dose of 500–750 mg/day for migraine, while higher doses may be necessary to treat epilepsy and mania effectively. Although some patients may respond to lower doses of preventive medications, if the therapeutic response is unsatisfactory and side effects are insignificant, increasing the dose may improve headache control. In general, each medication should be increased until headache control is achieved, unacceptable side effects develop, or the ceiling dose of the specific drug is reached and maintained for an adequate therapeutic trial.

A full therapeutic trial may take 2–6 months. In controlled clinical trials, efficacy is often first noted at 4 weeks and continues to increase for 3 months. It is not uncommon for a patient to be treated with a new preventive medication for 1–2 weeks and the treatment discontinued after the first breakthrough headache occurs. This practice ensures that preventive treatment will fail, as breakthrough headaches are almost inevitable during the dose-adjustment phase of treatment. The use of a headache diary can make trials of preventive medications much easier to interpret for physician and patient alike.

To obtain maximal benefit from preventive medication, the patient should not overuse analgesics, opioids, ergot derivatives, or triptans. In addition, oral contraceptives (OCs), hormonal replacement therapy, or vasodilating drugs, such as nifedipine or nitroglycerine, may interfere with preventive drugs.

Migraine headaches may improve with the passage of time, independent of treatment. If the headaches are well controlled, a drug holiday can

● **Table 6.22** *Choices of preventive treatment in migraine: influence of comorbid conditions*

Drug	Efficacy*	Side effects*	Comorbid condition	
			Relative contraindications	Relative indications
Beta-blockers	4+	2+	Asthma, depression, CHF, Raynaud's disease, diabetes	Hypertension, angina
Antiserotonin				
Pizotifen	3+	2+	Obesity	
Methysergide	4+	4+	Angina, PVD	Orthostatic hypotension
Calcium-channel blockers				
Verapamil	2+	1+	Constipation, hypotension	Migraine with aura, hypertension, angina, asthma
Flunarizine	4+	2+	Parkinson's disease	Hypertension, familial hemiplegic migraine
Antidepressants				
Tricyclic	4+	2+	Mania, urinary retention, heart block	Other pain disorders, depression, anxiety disorders, insomnia
SSRI	2+	1+	Mania	Depression, OCD
MAOI	4+	4+	Unreliable patient	Refractory depression
Anticonvulsants				
Valproate/divalproex	4+	2+	Liver disease, bleeding disorders	Mania, epilepsy, anxiety disorders
NSAID				
Naproxen	2+	2+	Ulcer disease, gastritis	Arthritis, other pain disorders
Other				
Riboflavin	2+	1+		Fear of drugs

*Ratings are on a scale from 1+ (lowest) to 4+ (highest).
CHF = congestive heart failure; OCD = obsessive compulsive disorder; PVD = peripheral vascular disease;
MAOI = monoamine oxidase inhibitor; SSRI = serotonin specific re-uptake inhibitor; NSAID = non-steroidal anti-inflammatory drug

be undertaken following a slow taper programme. Many patients experience continued relief after discontinuing the medication or they may not need the same dose. Dose reduction may provide a better risk-to-benefit ratio.

A woman with childbearing potential should be on adequate contraception before starting preventive or acute migraine medication. However, some women who are pregnant or who are attempting to become pregnant may still require preventive medications. If this is absolutely necessary, inform the patient and her partner of any potential risks and pick the medication with the least adverse effects on the fetus.

Medication

Beta-blockers

Since the relative efficacy of the different beta-blockers (propranolol, metoprolol, timolol, nadolol, and atenolol) has not been clearly estab-lished, choose a beta-blocker based on beta-selectivity, convenience of drug formulation, side effects, and the patient's individual reaction. We prefer nadolol and atenolol because of their long half-lives and favourable side-effect profiles, although propranolol remains a useful drug. Since beta-blockers can produce behavioural side effects, such as drowsiness, fatigue, lethargy, sleep disorders, nightmares, depression, memory disturbance, and hallucinations, we avoid them in patients with depression or low energy. Decreased exercise tolerance sometimes limits their use by athletes. Less common side effects include impotence, orthostatic hypotension, significant bradycardia, and aggravation of intrinsic muscle disease. We find beta-blockers especially useful in patients with angina or hypertension. They are relatively contraindicated in patients with congestive heart failure, asthma, Raynaud's disease, and insulin-dependent diabetes.

Antidepressants

We use both TCAs and selective serotonin reuptake inhibitors (SSRIs). The TCAs we use most commonly are nortriptyline and doxepin, and dothiepin (outside the United States), although only amitriptyline has demonstrated benefits in placebo-controlled, double-blind studies. We prefer TCAs for a patient with a sleep disturbance, as TCAs both prevent migraine and improve sleep. Similarly, we frequently use SSRIs, such as fluoxetine, paroxetine, and sertraline, based on their favourable side-effect profiles, although their efficacy in migraine prophylaxis has not been established. Fluoxetine has proved valuable in chronic daily headache (*see* Chapter 8).

Side effects of TCAs are common. Most involve antimuscarinic effects, such as dry mouth and sedation. The drugs also cause increased appetite and weight gain, and cardiac toxicity and orthostatic hypotension occur occasionally. Sexual dysfunction is not uncommon with SSRIs and can be treated with amantadine. Antidepressants are especially useful in patients with comorbid depression and anxiety disorders.

Calcium-channel blockers

Of the calcium-channel blockers available in the United States, verapamil is the only effective choice. This drug is especially useful in patients with hypertension or with contraindications to beta-blockers (such as asthma and Raynaud's disease). As the drug has an especially favourable side-effect profile, we use it preferentially for patients unlikely to tolerate cognitive side effects. We also use verapamil in patients with migraine who have prolonged aura or migrainous infarction. Constipation is verapamil's most common side effect. Flunarizine, the most effective drug of this class, is available in Europe and Canada but not in the United States. The symptoms of parkinsonism, produced by its antidopaminergic activity, as well as weight gain and drowsiness limit its use.

Anticonvulsant medications

Divalproex and valproate (in Europe) are very effective preventive medications for migraine. As demonstrated by four placebo-controlled studies, these drugs are effective in many patients at a low dose of 500–750 mg/day, although some patients require higher doses. In patients who do not respond to lower doses, we push the dose of valproate to a trough level of 120 mg/ml.

Side effects include sedation, hair loss, tremor, and changes in cognitive performance. Nausea, vomiting, and indigestion can occur, but these are self-limited side effects. While hepatotoxicity is the most serious side effect, irreversible hepatic dysfunction is extremely rare in adults. Baseline liver function studies should be obtained, but routine follow-up studies are probably not needed in adults on monotherapy. However, follow-up is necessary to adjust the dose and monitor side effects.

Valproate is especially useful when migraine occurs in patients who have comorbid epilepsy, anxiety disorders, or manic-depressive illness. The drug can be safely administered to patients with depression, Raynaud's disease, asthma, and diabetes, circumventing the contraindications to beta-blockers.

Serotonin antagonists

Methysergide was the first drug approved for migraine prevention and remains very effective. Side effects include transient muscle aching, claudication, abdominal cramps, nausea, weight gain, and hallucinations. Hallucinations are not uncommon after the first dose. The best-known complication of methysergide is the rare (1/2500) development of retroperitoneal, pulmonary, or endocardial fibrosis. The unreasonable fear of fibrotic complications limits its more widespread use. To prevent this complication, a drug holiday, which consists of a medication-free interval of 4 weeks following each 6-month course of continuous treatment, is recommended. We find methysergide to be a very effective drug with minimal side effects, but because of the need for a drug holiday we reserve its use to patients who have failed other treatment.

Cyproheptadine

Cyproheptadine is a 5-HT_{2A}, 5-HT_{2B}, and 5-HT_{2C} antagonist with antihistaminic and anticholinergic activity. It is often used for migraine prophylaxis in childhood migraine or hormonally mediated migraines. Open-label studies indicate that cyproheptadine improves migraine in 43–65% of patients, but comparative trials indicate that it is inferior to methysergide. Adverse drug reactions are considered to be less than those of methysergide and include drowsiness, dizziness, dry mouth, increased appetite, and weight gain. Cyproheptadine is contraindicated in patients with glaucoma. Administration of the majority of the dose at bedtime may minimize daytime drowsiness.

Pizotifen

Pizotifen is a benzocycloheptathiophene derivative structurally similar to cyproheptadine and the TCAs, and is available outside the United States. Pizotifen is a 5-HT$_2$ and histamine-1 antagonist with a long elimination half-life (about 23 hours) that can be given as a single evening dose, and has proved effective in placebo-controlled trials; side effects include drowsiness and increased appetite, with associated weight gain. Pizotifen is often used to treat adolescent migraineurs at doses of 0.5–1.5 mg daily, but adults may require up to 3 mg daily. Pizotifen has no known interaction with specific antimigraine compounds, such as ergotamine or the triptans.

Riboflavin

Riboflavin, (vitamin B$_2$) was recently shown to be effective in the treatment of migraine at a dose of 400 mg a day. Side effects are minimal, and it represents a scientifically proved, highly safe option for treatment.

Setting treatment priorities

The goals of treatment are to relieve or prevent the pain and associated symptoms of migraine and to optimize the patient's ability to function normally. We divide the preventive medications used to treat migraine into four major categories (Table 6.23):

- high-efficacy, relatively safe first-line treatments, which include beta-blockers, TCAs, pizotifen, and valproate;
- low to moderate-efficacy, relatively safe first-line treatments, which include SSRI, calcium-channel antagonists, NSAIDs, and riboflavin;
- high-efficacy second-line treatments (less safe or more difficult to use), which include methysergide and MAOIs; and
- second-line treatments of unproved or low efficacy, which include cyproheptadine and gabapentin.

When initiating preventive treatment, choose a drug from one of the first-line alternatives based on the patient's preferences and headache profile, the drug's side effects, and any coexisting or comorbid disease (see Table 6.12). Use the drug with the best risk-to-benefit ratio for the individual patient and take advantage of the drug's side-effect profile. Comorbid and coexistent diseases have important implications for treatment. The presence of a second illness provides therapeutic opportunities, but also imposes certain therapeutic limitations. In some instances, two or more conditions may be treated with a single drug. When migraine and hypertension and/or angina occur together, beta-blockers or calcium-channel blockers may be effective for all conditions. For the patient with migraine and depression, TCAs or SSRIs may be especially useful. For the patient with migraine and epilepsy or migraine and manic depressive illness, sodium valproate is the drug of choice. The pregnant migraineur who has a comorbid condition that requires treatment should be given a medication that is effective for both conditions and has the lowest potential for adverse effects on the fetus. In individuals with more than one disease, certain categories of treatment may be relatively contraindicated. For example, beta-blockers should be used with caution in the depressed migraineur; TCAs, neuroleptics, or sumatriptan may lower the seizure threshold and should be used with caution in the epileptic migraineur.

Drug combinations are commonly used for patients with refractory headache disorders. Some combinations, such as antidepressants and

● **Table 6.23** Preventive drugs

First-line choices	High efficacy:	Beta-blockers, tricyclic antidepressants, valproate verapami, pizotifen
	Low efficacy:	I, NSAID, SSRI, Riboflavin
Second-line choices	High efficacy:	Methysergide*
		Flunarizine
		MAOI*
	Unproven efficacy:	Cyproheptadine
		Gabapentin
		Lamotrigine

Significant adverse effects

beta-blockers, are suggested; others, such as beta-blockers and calcium-channel blockers, should be used with caution; and some, such as MAOIs and SSRIs, are contraindicated because of potentially lethal interactions (Table 6.24). Many clinicians find that the combination of an anti-depressant (such as a TCA or SSRI) and a beta-blocker is synergistic. Valproate, used in combination with antidepressants, is a logical choice to treat refractory migraine that is com-plicated by depression or bipolar disease.

Use of abortive medication in patients on preventive treatment

Preventive medication is considered effective if it decreases the frequency of attacks by more than 50% in more than 50% of treated patients. Preventive medication may also decrease the intensity and duration of attacks, and may make abortive medications more effective. Using pre-ventive and abortive medications together pre-sents a new set of complexities:

- the amount of acute medication must be limited to prevent the development of drug-induced daily rebound headache and loss of efficacy of the preventive medication; and
- certain acute medications should be used with caution, or not at all, when certain preventive medications are used (Table 6.25).

For example, for a patient on methysergide, each of ergotamine, DHE, and sumatriptan potentially could have enhanced vasoconstrictive properties. However, many authorities have found that the ergots are more effective in patients treated with methysergide. Since MAOIs inhibit the metabolism of sumatriptan, increasing its half-life and there-fore the patient's exposure to the drug, the dose of oral sumatriptan should be reduced and used cautiously, if at all, in patients who take MAOIs. Meperidine and sympathomimetics are potentially lethal additions to an MAOI and may result in serotonin syndrome or hypertensive crisis.

Status migrainosus

Status migrainosus is a condition characterized by severe, persistent headache that is often associated

● **Table 6.24** Drug combination

Suggested	Antidepressant	Beta-blocker
		Calcium-channel blocker
		Valproate
		Methysergide
	Methysergide	Calcium-channel blocker
	SSRI	Tricyclic antidepressant
Caution	Beta-blocker	Calcium-channel blocker
		Methysergide
	MAOI	Amitriptyline or nortriptyline
Contrain-dications	MAOI	SSRI
		Most tricyclic antidepressants (except amitriptyline or nortriptyline)
		Carbamazepine

with intractable nausea and vomiting. Prior to instituting treatment, serious organic causes of headache must be excluded. We start treatment by rehydrating the patient with intravenous fluids and using one of the treatment options in Table 6.26. If the headache persists and is associated with intractable nausea and vomiting, hospital admis-sion may be required. Some indications for admis-sion are listed in Table 6.27. Various treatment options have been explored for type of headache and include referral to a neurologist or headache expert. Intravenous chlorpromazine, droperidol, and prochlorperazine control intractable headache effectively. Although neuroleptics may be locally irritating when given intravenously, they are prob-ably more effective than when given intramuscu-larly or by suppository. We have found that

● **Table 6.25** Cautions in acute medication use

Agent	Caution	Contraindicated
Methysergide	Ergotamine, dihydroergotamine, 5-HT$_1$ agonists	
Monoamine oxidase inhibitors	Oral sumatriptan	Pethidine (meperidine)
		Sympathomimetics (isometheptene)
Non-steroidal anti-inflammatory drugs	Other NSAIDs or aspirin-containing compounds	
Valproate	Overuse of short-acting barbiturates	

droperidol (2.5 mg), haloperidol (5 mg), and thio-thixene (5 mg) given intramuscularly are effective as adjunct or primary treatment for the severe migraine headache. Intravenous haloperidol has recently been used successfully.

Intravenous prochlorperazine 5 mg followed by intravenous DHE is a safe and effective means of terminating a migraine attack. The combination of intravenous metoclopramide and intravenous DHE is more effective in treating an acute migraine attack than is intramuscular meperidine. Prochlorperazine

(10 mg, 2 ml) and DHE (1 mg, 1 ml) can be mixed in a syringe and 2 cm^3 of the mixture injected intra-venously. If the headache is not relieved in 15–30 minutes, the remainder of the dose can be injected. At times, the addition of 5–10 mg of intravenous diazepam terminates the headache attack.

Repetitive intravenous dihydroergotamine
Patients who have truly intractable headaches should be admitted to the hospital. A neurological consultation is obtained and the patient treated with repeated doses of intravenous DHE. The patient should be pre-treated with metoclopramide 10 mg i.v. and then DHE 0.5 mg (Figure 6.16). If the patient has no nausea and the headache persists, another 0.5 mg DHE is given. If the patient's

---

● **Table 6.26** *Treatment of status migrainosus*

- Start intravenous fluids
- Pretreat with prochlorperazine 5–10 mg i.v. or metoclopramide 10 mg i.v.
- Treat with dihydroergotamine 0.5–1 mg i.v.
- If headache persists after 1 h give additional 0.5 mg dihydroergotamine i.v.
- Additions: dexamethasone 4 mg i.v.; diazepam 5–10 mg i.v.
- Alternatives:
  ketorolac 30–60 mg i.m.
  narcotics
  chlorpromazine 0.1 mg/kg

● **Table 6.27** *Indications for admission to hospital*

Emergency or urgent admission*

- Migraine variants such as hemiplegic migraine.
- Suspected CNS infection.
- Acute vascular disorder.
- Drug toxicity.
- Status migrainosus.
- Failed outpatient treatment of severe headache.

Non-emergent admission

- Headache causing interruption and compromise of the ability to carry out activities of daily living.
- Chronic daily refractory headache or cluster headache that does not respond to aggressive outpatient treatment.
- Headache complicated by significant depression or psychiatric disturbance.
- Headache accompanied by significant medical or surgical problem.
- Headache treatment requiring polypharmacy with potentially dangerous drug interactions or requiring close observation during initiation (MOAIs).
- Headache complicated by drug overuse that could not be safely or effectively treated overnight.

* *Diagnosis itself warrants admission*

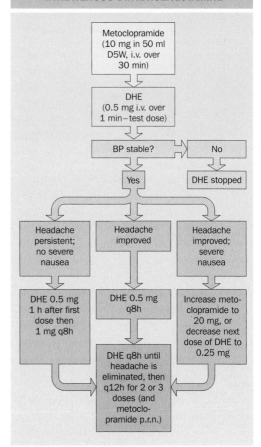

INTRAVENOUS DIHYDROERGOTAMINE

● **Figure 6.16** *Treatment protocol of repetitive intravenous dihydroergotamine. (D5W = dextrose 5% in water.)*

headache is gone, 1 mg DHE is continued every 8 hours. If nausea develops, the dose of DHE is decreased and the metoclopramide increased. Metoclopramide can cause dyskinesia and patients may complain of restlessness, which can be controlled with diphenhydramine 50 mg i.v. Both drugs are continued as needed, the DHE every 8 hours until the patient is headache free, at which time it is tapered and discontinued. Although the American Academy of Neurology found it safe to use repetitive intravenous DHE for up to 7 days, we usually, but not always, limit its use to 4–5 days.

If the patient does not start to improve within 2–3 days, we change our treatment approach. Other treatment options include the repetitive use of intravenous neuroleptics (prochlorperazine 5–10 mg i.v. every 8 hours, chlorpromazine 10–25 mg every 8 hours, droperidol 1–2.5 mg i.v. every 6–8 hours), and/or intravenous corticosteroids (dexamethasone 4 mg or methylprednisolone 200 mg).

Menstrual migraine

Migraine is often associated with menstruation and may be refractory to treatment. When migraine occurs before menstruation, it is sometimes associated with premenstrual syndrome

● **Table 6.28** *Premenstrual syndrome*

Depression	Backache
Anxiety	Breast tenderness
Crying spells	Swelling
Difficulty in thinking	Nausea
Lethargy	

(PMS; Table 6.28). When migraine occurs during menstruation, it is often associated with dysmenorrhoea. It is important to determine when the attacks occur because medications that are effective for migraine related to dysmenorrhoea may not help headache associated with PMS. A headache calendar can help establish a relationship between headache and the menstrual cycle. Based on clinical experience, the frequency of menstrual migraine is reported to be 60–70%.

Most women have an increase in headache attacks at the time of menses (Figure 6.17), but some women have migraine (usually without aura) only with menses. Menstrual migraine can be defined as attacks triggered by menstruation on a regular basis and occurring 1–2 days before and up to 3 days after menses (Table 6.29). Menstrual migraine is triggered by falling oestrogen levels (Figure 6.18).

Women who have headache throughout their menstrual cycle should be treated with reassurance,

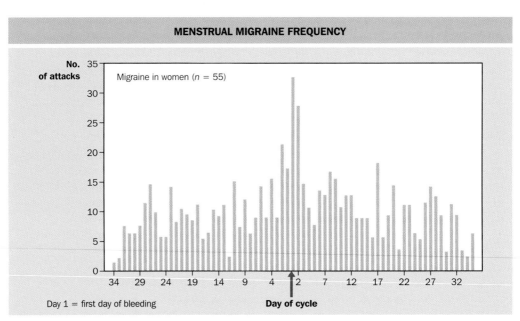

● **Figure 6.17** *Menstrual migraine frequency. (Adapted from MacGregor et al., 1990.)*

HORMONAL FLUCTUATIONS DURING THE MENSTRUAL CYCLE

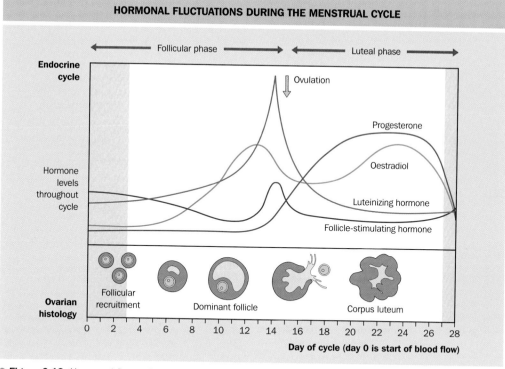

● **Figure 6.18** *Hormonal fluctuations during the menstrual cycle.*

● **Table 6.29** *Menstrual migraine definition*

Premenstrual migraine	Menstrual migraine
Attacks occur −7 to −2 days*	Attacks occur −1 to +4 days*
* Day 0 = onset of menses	

● **Table 6.30** *Treatment of menstrual migraine*

- Non-steroidal anti-inflammatory drugs
- Ergotamine and its derivatives
- Perimenstrual use of standard prophylactic drugs
- Short course of corticosteroids or major tranquillizers
- Hormonal therapy
  Oestrogens (with or without androgens or progestogen)
  Synthetic androgens (danazol)
  Anti-oestrogen (tamoxifen)
  Dopamine agonists (bromocriptine)

education, and pharmacological intervention. Behavioural intervention may be useful in selected instances. Menstrual migraine differs from non-menstrual migraine in that the former is not associated with an aura and is of longer duration, and there may be more headache recurrence after treatment (Table 6.30).

Drugs that have proved effective or are commonly used for the acute treatment of menstrual migraine include NSAIDs, DHE, the triptans, and the combination of aspirin, paracetamol, and caffeine. Prostaglandin production may be enhanced in menstrual migraine. The effectiveness of the NSAID may result from blocking prostaglandin synthesis by inhibiting the enzyme cyclooxygenase; NSAIDs must be used in adequate doses.

A non-selective 5-HT$_1$ agonist, DHE is available in parenteral form and as a nasal spray, and is effective for the treatment of menstrual migraine. In an open study, patients with menstrual migraine responded as well to 1 mg i.m. of DHE as did patients with non-menstrual migraine. Headache, nausea, and vomiting were all well controlled. Sumatriptan, zolmitriptan, and rizatriptan are as effective for migraine related to menstruation as for migraine not related to menstruation, and, in addition, these drugs control the nausea and vomiting associated with attacks.

If severe menstrual migraine cannot be controlled with NSAIDs, ergots, DHE, or the triptans, then analgesics in combination with opioids, high-dose corticosteroids, major tranquillizers (chlorpromazine, haloperidol, thiothixene), or repetitive intravenous DHE can be tried. Women with frequent, severe menstrual migraine are candidates for preventive therapy (either continuous or short term) and often respond better to acute therapy when on preventive treatment (Table 6.31). If these fail, a trial of hormonal therapy may be indicated.

The goal of standard, continuous, preventive therapy is to reduce the frequency, duration, and intensity of attacks. Preventive therapy may eliminate all headaches except those associated with menses. Women using preventive medication who continue to have menstrual migraine can increase the dose of their medication prior to their menses. An alternative strategy is short-term prophylaxis during a defined period of increased vulnerability. Since menstrual migraine typically occurs at the same time of month or in association with symptoms that herald its occurrence, the timed use of medications is appropriate. Women who do not use preventive medicine or who have migraine exclusively with their menses can be treated perimenstrually with short-term prophylaxis. Treatment of coexistent PMS may help control premenstrual headache. Drugs that have been used for short-term prophylaxis include NSAIDs, ergotamine, DHE, methysergide, methylergonovine maleate, the triptans, and magnesium. In adequate doses, NSAIDs can be used preventively 1 or 2 days before the expected onset of headache and continued for the duration of vulnerability. If the first NSAID fails, a different NSAID from another chemical class should be tried (Figure 6.19).

Ergotamine and DHE can be used for short-term prophylaxis without a significant risk of ergot dependence. Ergotamine tartrate at bedtime or twice a day is an effective prophylactic agent. Ergotamine in combination with belladonna and phenobarbital may be useful in treating other perimenstrual symptoms in addition to headache. Given every 8 hours for 6 days, beginning 3 days before the expected onset of headache, DHE nasal spray was more effective than placebo in a double-blind, short-term trial for the treatment of

● **Table 6.31** *Preventive treatment of menstrual migraine*

Perimenstrual use of standard preventive drugs
Perimenstrual use of non-standard preventive drugs
Non-steroidal anti-inflammatory drugs
Ergotamine and its derivatives
Triptans
Magnesium
Hormonal therapy
Oestrogens (with or without androgens or progestin)
Combined oral contraceptives
Synthetic androgens (danazol)
Anti-oestrogen (tamoxifen)
Medical oophorectomy (GnRH analogues)
Dopamine agonists
Bromocriptine

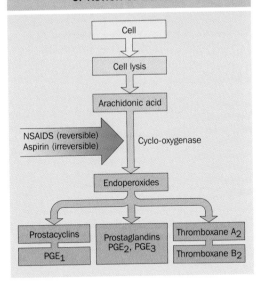

● **Figure 6.19** *Prostaglandins and the mechanism of action of NSAIDs.*

menstrual migraine. Oral sumatriptan (25 mg three times daily) given 2–3 days before the expected headache onset and continued for a total of 5 days was effective in an open-label study of menstrual migraine. Oral magnesium (360 mg of magnesium pyrrolidone carboxylic acid) decreases the severity of PMS symptoms and the duration and intensity of menstrual migraine that occurs prior to the onset of menstruation.

Popular but ineffective treatments for menstrual migraine include diuretics and vitamins. Diuretics help with fluid retention, but not with menstrual migraine. The efficacy of pyridoxine to treat both PMS and menstrual migraine has not been proved in double-blind studies. In fact, high doses of pyridoxine have been reported to cause a sensory neuropathy.

If severe menstrual migraine cannot be controlled by these measures, hormonal therapy may be indicated. Successful hormonal or hormonal modulation therapy for menstrual migraine has been reported using oestrogens, combined OCs, synthetic androgens, selective oestrogen receptor modulators (SERMS) and antagonists, and medical oophorectomy with gonadotropin-releasing hormone (GnRH) analogues.

The decrease in oestrogen levels during the late luteal phase of the menstrual cycle is a trigger for migraine. Oestrogen replacement prior to menstruation has been used to prevent migraine. The oestradiol cutaneous patch provides a relatively stable plasma-oestrogen level over the time of application. Serum oestrogen levels rise within 4 hours of applying the transdermal patch, are proportional to the dose, and require at least an oestradiol transdermal system in a patch dose of at least 100 μg/day to be effective. Combinations of oestrogens and progestogens or progestogens alone in the form of OCs may be a reasonable approach for some patients with intractable menstrual migraine, particularly if the headache is associated with severe dysmenorrhoea. Women on OCs who have menstrual-related problems can extend the active OCs for 6–12 weeks and delay the symptoms related to menstruation.

Specialists may use danazol (which is an androgen derivative), tamoxifen (SERM), and bromocriptine for short-term perimenstrual treatment.

Neither hysterectomy nor oophorectomy has proved effective in migraine treatment. However, medical ovariectomy using GnRH analogues to suppress ovulation are effective in refractory PMS. Some physicians are again advocating the use of hysterectomy and oophorectomy in women with severe intractable PMS or menstrual migraine who respond to medical ovariectomy. No long-term follow-up or controlled studies are underway to prove the effectiveness of this radical procedure.

Migraine in the menopause

Menopause presents a particular set of problems for women with migraine. Although migraine prevalence decreases in the mid-to-late 40s, an individual's attacks may worsen at menopause. One study showed that two-thirds of women with prior migraine improved with physiological menopause. In contrast, surgical menopause resulted in a worsening of migraine in two-thirds of women with prior migraine. Other studies have shown that hysterectomy or oophorectomy is not effective treatment for migraine at any age despite recent suggestions to the contrary. Oestrogen replacement therapy can exacerbate migraine or, alone or with testosterone, can relieve it. The use of drugs for treatment of migraine in menopausal women who do not need replacement oestrogens should be guided by their cardiac and renal status. Refractory cases may be treated with hormonal replacement.

Headache management can be difficult in women who require oestrogen replacement therapy for menopausal symptoms but who develop headaches as a result of the therapy. Several empirical strategies may be utilized, as described in Table 6.32. Consultation with a gynaecologist

● **Table 6.32** *Treatment of hormonal replacement headache*

Oestrogens
Reduce oestrogen dose
Change oestrogen type from conjugated oestrogen to pure oestradiol to synthetic oestrogen to pure oestrone
Convert from interrupted into continuous dosing
Convert from oral into parenteral dosing
Add androgens
Switch to selective oestrogen-receptor modulator

Progestin
Switch from interrupted (cyclic) to continuous lower dose
Change progestin type
Change delivery system (p.o. to vaginal)
Discontinue progestin (periodic endometrial biopsy or vaginal ultrasound)

and a headache specialist may be indicated because of the intractable nature of this problem.

Migraine associated with oral contraceptive use

The various oral contraceptive preparations are listed in Table 6.33. Hormonal contraceptive steroids are available as oral preparations (OCs), subcutaneous implants, and depo-injections. There are three major types of OC formulations: fixed-dose combinations, phasic combinations, and progestin only. Formulations with 50 μg or more of oestrogen are now called first-generation OCs, those with less than 50 μg of oestrogen are called second-generation OCs, and formulations with the new progestins (desogestrel, norgestimate, and gestodene) are called third-generation OCs.

Persistent controversy exists concerning OCs and the risk of stroke in migraineurs. The incidence of ischaemic stroke is low in women of reproductive age, and any risk attributable to OC use is small. Migraine itself may be a risk factor for stroke in women under 45 years of age. Migraine with aura may have twice the risk of migraine without aura. The risk for stroke is higher in women over the age of 35 years, and OCs should be used with caution in these women, particularly when other risk factors are present. The risk of stroke can be reduced if users are younger than 35 years of age, do not smoke, do not have a history of hypertension, and have blood pressure measured before the start of OC use. A positive interaction between OCs, smoking, and stroke exists. Current OC preparations, including those that contain the newest progestogens, are associated with a lower risk of cardiovascular disease relative to the risk associated with the original high-dose oestrogen contraceptives and the risk associated with full-term pregnancy. Cardiovascular disease occurs mainly among OC users who smoke or have other risk factors.

Contraceptive use

The older combined OCs can induce, change, or alleviate headaches. The first migraine attack can be triggered by OCs, most often in women with a family history of migraine. Existing migraine

● **Table 6.33** Oral contraceptives

Type	Progestin (mg)/ethinyl oestradiol (mg)
Combination monophasic	
Second generation	
Ethynodiol diacetate	1/30,1/35,1/50
Levonorgestrel	0.1/20, 0.15/30
Norethindrone	0.4/35, 0.5/35, 1/20, 1/35, 1/50
Norethindrone acetate	1.5/30
Norgestrel	0.3/30, 0.5/50
Third generation	
Desogestrel	0.15/30
Norgestimate	0.25/35
Biphasic	
Norethindrone	0.5/35 and 1/35
Triphasic	
Norethindrone	1/20, 1/30, 1/35,.5/35,.75/35, 1/35,.5/35, 1/35,.5/35
Levonorgestrel	0.05/30,.075/40,.125/30
Norgestimate	0.18/35, 0.215/35, 0.25/35
Progestin only	
Norethindrone	0.35
Norgestrel	0.075

may exacerbate and headaches may occur on the days off the OC. The headache pattern may become more severe and frequent and may be associated with neurological symptoms. In most women, however, the headache pattern does not change, and some women may have a distinct improvement in their headaches. New onset of migraine usually occurs in the early cycles of OC use, but it can occur after prolonged OC usage. Stopping the OC may not bring immediate headache relief; there may be a delay of 0.5–1 year, or there may be no improvement.

Hormonal contraception may generate new headaches or aggravate or even ameliorate preexisting headaches. The risks and benefits of different types of contraception, including hormonal contraception, should be discussed with the patient. Women who take OCs must be followed for headache aggravation or neurological symptoms. Women should not use OCs if they smoke or have uncontrolled hypertension or other cardiovascular disease (such as thromboembolism, thrombophlebitis, stroke, vasculitis, or diabetes with retinopathy) or nephropathy. Progestins can be used for contraception when oestrogens have caused increased headaches or are contraindicated.

The use of OCs is relatively safe for women with migraine who do not have aura and are less than 35 years of age. Women with intractable menstrual migraine or a history of headache relief with OCs are particularly good candidates for a trial of OC. Although OC use for women with migraine who have typical aura and who are under 35 years of age is probably safe, caution is required. We believe that OCs should not be used in women with hemiplegic, basilar, confusional migraine, or prolonged aura. Start with a formulation of less than 50 μg of ethinyl oestradiol. Use formulations with the lowest androgenic potency of progestin; progestin-only formulations have a lower incidence of adverse metabolic effects than do the combination formulations. Women whose headaches increase when they start on a combination OC, but who want to continue OC, should consider switching to a lower oestrogen dose preparation with a different progestin.

Summary

- Physical and neurological examination and laboratory studies for migraine are usually normal, thus serving to exclude other, more ominous, causes of headache. Migraine headache is diagnosed based on retrospective reporting.
- Migraine attacks have three phases – premonitory (prodrome), attack proper (headache with or without aura), and headache resolution. The type and quality of migraine attacks vary among individuals and within the same individual.
- Effective migraine treatment includes accurate diagnosis, explanation to the patient, a treatment plan, and setting priorities.
- Comorbid disease presents therapeutic opportunities and limitations.
- Acute medications include analgesics, antiemetics, anxiolytics, NSAIDs, ergots, corticosteroids, major tranquillizers, opioids, and triptans (selective 5-HT$_1$ agonists). Overuse of acute drugs may result in rebound headache.
- Preventive medications include beta-blockers, calcium-channel blockers, antidepressants, serotonin antagonists, anticonvulsants, and NSAIDs.
- Menstrual migraine occurs at the time of the greatest fluctuation in oestrogen levels. Hysterectomy and oophorectomy are not effective in treating migraine.
- Although migraine prevalence decreases with advancing age, it can regress or worsen at menopause.

Further reading

Adler CS, Adler SM, Friedman AP. A historical perspective on psychiatric thinking about headache. In: Adler CS, Adler SM, Packard RC (eds). *Psychiatric Aspects of Headache.* Baltimore: Williams and Wilkins, 1987: 3–21.

Ferrari MD, Haan J. Drug treatment of migraine attacks. In: Goadsby PJ, Silberstein SD (eds). *Blue Books of Practical Neurology (Headache).* Boston: Butterworth–Heinemann, 1997: 117–30.

Giammarco R, Edmeads J, Dodick D. *Critical Decisions in Headache Management.* BC Decker Inc., Hamilton, 1998.

Hutchinson M, O'Riordan J, Javed M et al. Familial hemiplegic migraine and autosomal dominant arteriopathy with leukoencephalopathy. *Ann Neurol* 1995; 38: 817–24.

Lance JW. Preventive treatment in migraine. In: Goadsby PJ, Silberstein SD (eds). *Blue Books of Practical Neurology (Headache).* Boston: Butterworth–Heinemann, 1997: 131–42.

Lance JW, Goadsby PJ. *Mechanism and Management of Headache.* London: Butterworth–Heinemann, 1998.

MacGregor EA et al. Migraine and menstruation. *Cephalalgia* 190; 10: 305.

Sacks O. *Migraine – Understanding a Common Disorder.* University of California Press, 1985.

Silberstein SD. Migraine symptoms: results of a survey of self-reported migraineurs. *Headache* 1995; 35: 387–96.

Silberstein SD, Lipton RB. Overview of diagnosis and treatment of migraine. *Neurology* 1994; 44(7) :6–16.

Silberstein SD, Merriam GR. Sex hormones and headache. In: Goadsby PJ, Silberstein SD (eds). *Blue Books of Practical Neurology (Headache).* Boston: Butterworth–Heinemann, 1997: 143–76.

Silberstein SD, Saper J. Migraine: diagnosis and treatment. In: Delessio D, Silberstein SD (eds). *Wolff's Headache and Other Head Pain*, 6th edn. New York: Oxford University Press, 1993: 96–170.

Silberstein SD, Lipton RB, Goadsby P. *Headache in Clinical Practice.* Oxford: Isis Medical Media, 1998.

Spierings ELH. Symptomatology and pathogenesis. In: Spierings ELH (ed.), *Management of Migraine.* Newton: Butterworth–Heinemann, 1996: 7–19.

Fisher CM. *Late life migraine accompaniments: further experience.* Stroke 1986; 17: 1033–42.

Saper JR, Silberstein SD, Gordon CD, Hamel RL. *Handbook of Headache Management.* Baltimore: Williams and Wilkins, 1993.

7 Tension-type headache: diagnosis and treatment

Introduction

Tension-type headache (TTH), the most common headache type, is classified as either episodic or chronic based on the frequency and duration of the attacks (Table 7.1). Scalp tenderness and increased electromyographic (EMG) activity of the pericranial muscles, often a feature of TTH, lead to the term 'muscle contraction' headaches. As it became clear that excessive muscle contraction also occurs in migraine, the simple muscle contraction hypothesis fell out of favour. The term 'tension headache' was adopted to suggest that psychological tension was the cause of the disorder. Currently, it is not clear that either hypothesis is correct. The term 'tension-type headache' was introduced to overcome this confusion, while leaving some historical link to the terminology that was previously used. The term is not ideal, but it does reflect a loose consensus about the condition, which is an extraordinarily common disorder.

The lifetime period prevalence of episodic TTH (ETTH) in Denmark is 69% in men and 88% in women, and in the past year 63% of men and 88% of women had at least one TTH. United States prevalence estimates are closer to 40% in both women and men and increases with education. In population-based studies in both the United States and Spain, the prevalence of frequent headache (i.e. one that occurs more than 15 days/month) is about 4.5%. Chronic TTH (CTTH) is the most common type of frequent headache in the population, accounting for about two-thirds of frequent headaches; it shows a more striking female preponderance (1.9:1), intermediate between ETTH and migraine. The relationship of CTTH and socioeconomic status is also intermediate between those of ETTH and migraine. Women are slightly more likely to be affected than men, but the gender ratio is not as great as that of migraine. Also, TTH is common at all ages, including childhood and adolescence.

This chapter begins with definitions and clinical characteristics of TTH. The pathogenesis is

● **Table 7.1** *Tension-type headache (IHS)*

2.1	**Episodic tension-type headache**
	Diagnostic criteria:
A	At least 10 previous headache episodes fulfilling criteria B–D listed below. Number of days with such headache <180/year (<15/month).
B	Headache lasting from 30 minutes to 7 days.
C	At least two of the following pain characteristics: 1 Pressing/tightening (non-pulsating) quality. 2 Mild or moderate intensity (may inhibit, but does not prohibit activities). 3 Bilateral location. 4 No aggravation by walking stairs or similar routine physical activity.
D	Both of the following: 1 No nausea or vomiting (anorexia may occur). 2 Photophobia and phonophobia are absent, one but not the other is present.
2.1.1	**Episodic tension-type headache associated with disorder of pericranial muscles**
	Diagnostic criteria:
A	Fulfills criteria for 2.1.
B	At least one of the following: 1 Increased tenderness of pericranial muscles. 2 Increased EMG level of pericranial muscles.
2.1.2	**Episodic tension-type headache unassociated with disorder of pericranial muscles**
	Diagnostic criteria:
A	Fulfills criteria for 2.1.
B	No increased tenderness or EMG activity of pericranial muscles.
2.2	**Chronic tension-type headache**
	Diagnostic criteria:
A	Average headache frequency >15 days/month (180 days/year) for >6 months fulfilling criteria B–D.
B	At least two of the following pain characteristics: 1 Pressing/tightening quality. 2 Mild or moderate severity (may inhibit but does not prohibit activities). 3 Bilateral location. 4 No aggravation by walking stairs or similar routine physical activity.
C	Both of the following: 1 No vomiting. 2 No more than one of the following: nausea, photophobia, or phonophobia.
2.2.1	**Chronic tension-type headache associated with disorder of pericranial muscles**
2.2.2	**Chronic tension-type headache unassociated with disorder of pericranial muscles**

reviewed, treatment described, and finally the relationship of TTH to migraine is discussed.

Definition and clinical characteristics

The spectrum of severity of TTH is wide, varying from rare, brief episodes to frequent, often continuous, disabling headaches. Definition of ETTH is given by the International Headache Society (IHS) diagnostic criteria listed in Table 7.1. The criteria establish a sharp contrast with migraine, as discussed below. For CTTH, the patient must experience head pain for at least 15 days a month for at least 6 months; many patients with CTTH have headaches almost every day. In comparison with patients who have ETTH, patients with CTTH have more disability, are more difficult to treat, and are more likely to overuse acute headache medication.

The following signs and symptoms help identify TTH:

- prodrome and aura are absent;
- pain is usually mild to moderate in intensity (in contrast to the moderate-to-severe pain of migraine);
- most patients have bilateral pain, although 10–20% of patients experience unilateral pain;
- pain location varies (frontal, temporal, occipital, or parietal regions are affected, alone or in combination, with frontal and temporal pain being the most common) – the patient sometimes describes a hatband pattern of pain;
- some patients have neck or jaw discomfort or problems with the temporomandibular joint (e.g. the presence of reciprocal clicking of the temporomandibular joint or pain with maximum jaw opening and pain upon palpation are sensitive clinical signs of oromandibular dysfunction);
- some patients may have tender spots and palpable nodules in the pericranial or cervical muscles (trigger points);
- besides headache, other features are generally absent (most patients lack the associated symptoms of migraine, but some report slight photophobia, phonophobia, or nausea);
- TTH can interfere with daily activity, but on average individual attacks produce less disability than does migraine; and
- routine physical activity rarely influences headache intensity (in contrast with migraine).

The contrasts between migraine and TTH are sharp. Migraine pain is unilateral; TTH pain is bilateral. Migraine pain is throbbing; TTH is a steady ache. Migraine pain is moderate to severe in intensity; TTH pain is mild to moderate. Migraine requires the presence of nausea or vomiting or photophobia and phonophobia, features rare in TTH. Aura is only required to make the diagnosis of migraine with aura (classic migraine).

Differential diagnosis

Like the other primary headaches, no diagnostic tests are available for TTH. Diagnosis requires the exclusion of other primary and secondary headache disorders and the identification of a characteristic clinical profile. The diagnosis of TTH is clinical, based on the history, as well as a normal general and neurological examination. While the pain profile of TTH is characteristic (bilateral, mild-to-moderate, pressing pain), the associated symptoms are diagnostic based on their absence. Specifically, nausea, photophobia, and phonophobia are virtually absent, although in ETTH either phonophobia or photophobia may occur; in CTTH, any of the three can occur. The physician must be alert for atypical symptoms or abnormalities on neurological examination, because patients with secondary headaches often have a headache profile that mimics TTH. For example, brain tumour headache often begins as a bilateral pressure pain with few associated symptoms. High- and low-pressure syndromes and hemicrania continua also enter into the differential diagnosis.

Precipitating factors

Often, TTH begins in the afternoon, during a stressful workday. Lack of sleep is also a common precipitating factor. In one study, 39% of healthy volunteers developed TTH after sleep deprivation.

Other studies show that TTH sufferers may have more problems with sleep than do migraineurs or non-headache control subjects. Eyestrain, sitting in uncomfortable positions, bad posture, and stress may cause TTH in susceptible individuals. Precipitating factors are better characterized for migraine than for TTH.

Episodic tension-type headache and migraine

Migraine and ETTH have traditionally been considered distinct entities, separation codified by the 1988 IHS headache classification. In the IHS system, if a patient has more than one type of headache, each type needs to be diagnosed. Thus, many patients are diagnosed as having both migraine and TTH. Some believe that migraine and TTH are related entities that differ more in severity than kind. This presumes that all TTH is one problem, which is far from clear. Both migraine and TTH are 'benign recurring headaches that occur in the headache-prone'. Some patients, and indeed families, seem headache-prone in the sense that they have frequent migraine and TTH triggered in situations that non-headache patients would find innocuous. Migraine and TTH occur together more frequently than would be expected by chance. Most migraineurs (62%) also have TTH, and 25% of TTH patients also have migraine. The clinical syndrome of TTH may result from two distinct mechanisms. In migraineurs, it may be an expression of mild migraine. In non-migraineurs, pure TTH may be a distinct disorder not related to migraine. We believe that in individuals with migraine some headaches that resemble TTH in their clinical features may arise from migraine-like mechanisms and respond to triptans. In individuals without any migrainous features, pure ETTH appears not to respond to triptans, supporting the distinction between the disorders. This general principle can be useful in clinical practice, since it suggests that in the headache-prone patients, medicines (particularly preventive agents) may be useful for both types of headache.

Chronic tension-type headache

The primary difference between CTTH and ETTH is attack frequency. By definition, CTTH attacks occur 15 or more days per month for at least 6 months. The pain criteria for CTTH and ETTH are

the same. However, CTTH allows the associated features of nausea but not vomiting, or either photophobia or phonophobia occurring alone. This distinction is somewhat artificial and can be set aside in clinical practice without penalty.

However, CTTH must be distinguished from other varieties of chronic daily headache (CDH), including transformed migraine. In their pure episodic forms, migraine and TTH are easily distinguished, but as migraine headache frequency increases, the clinical distinctions become blurred. For some patients, as the course of migraine progresses, the headaches increase in frequency and decrease in severity, and the associated migrainous features decline in prominence. Among patients with transformed migraine, the headaches, which occur on a daily or near-daily basis, often come to resemble those of CTTH, with bilateral pressure pain and little nausea, photophobia, or phonophobia. Superimposed on these background headaches may be occasional full-blown migraine attacks. The IHS system currently recommends assigning two diagnoses to these patients – migraine and CTTH. We advocate distinguishing two clinical syndromes, transformed migraine and CTTH (see Chapter 8).

Mechanisms of tension-type headache

It was thought that TTH arose from sustained muscle contraction, perhaps as a consequence of emotion or tension. However, there is no relationship between muscle contraction, tenderness, and the location of headache. Various evidence suggests that migraine and TTH have a similar pathogenesis – both are associated with muscle tenderness, an abnormal electromyogram, abnormal electrophysiological profiles, exteroceptive suppression (ES2; a measure of brainstem pain modulation), abnormal platelet serotonin, and (when headaches are severe and chronic) decreased cerebrospinal fluid β-endorphin, an endogenous opioid. Studies indicate that patients with ETTH, CTTH, and migraine have increased EMG activity in some muscles when multiple muscles are sampled under different conditions. However, no increase in neck muscle EMG activity was found in one study during continuous monitoring by ambulatory electromyogram during a headache attack. No significant association has been found between increased EMG activity and pericranial tenderness. Pain sensitivity may be increased in some TTH patients.

TTH is now believed to result from abnormal neuronal sensitivity and pain facilitation, not abnormal muscle contraction:

- pain sensitivity is increased;
- tenderness is increased in some pericranial muscles under some conditions independent of headache; and
- tenderness and increased EMG activity vary independently.

Thus, headache is not directly related to muscle contraction and focal tenderness. In migraine and CTTH, there may be hypersensitivity of neurons in the trigeminal nucleus caudalis, which is the major relay nucleus for head and face pain. The trigeminal nucleus caudalis receives pain input from cephalic blood vessels and pericranial muscles, and dual supraspinal input, both inhibitory and facilitatory. Many studies of the mechanisms of headache pain indicate that tenderness, not muscle contraction, correlates with headache development. Tenderness may have a central cause or it may result from muscle contraction that results in activation and chemical sensitization on myofascial mechanoreceptors and/or their afferent fibres. The therapeutic approaches to headache should consider the importance of peripheral and central mechanisms, since they may vary and produce complex interactions.

Fibromyalgia, myofascial pain syndrome, tension myalgia, and tension-type headache

Fibromyalgia is a chronic disorder, characterized by widespread pain and musculoskeletal tenderness throughout the body, that mainly affects women (90%). Associated symptoms include sleep disturbance (75%), morning stiffness (77%), fatigue (81%), paraesthesias, headache (52.8%), and anxiety (47.8%) or depression (31.5%). Since it is associated with a decreased pain threshold, pain from other disorders, such as headache, may be exacerbated.

Myofascial pain syndrome is distinguished from fibromyalgia by being a focal disorder associated with trigger points. The patient with myofascial pain has focal or regional complaints. Both fibromyalgia and TTH may have tender spots, relief with trigger point injection, and, when chronic, associated anxiety and depression. There may also be increased pain sensitivity and involvement of the pain control systems, which suggests that TTH may overlap with localized fibromyalgia of the pericranial structures.

Relationship to depression

Although many have attempted to portray ETTH as a primary psychological disorder, no evidence of associated anxiety or depression has been found, in contrast to the frequent association of anxiety and depression found with migraine and the psychological distress found with CDH (described in Chapter 8). However, some investigators believe that CTTH can mask depression or other serious emotional disorders. A persistent, vague headache for which no organic cause can be determined is frequently blamed on underlying psychic distress. Martin *et al.*, in a study that did not have adequate controls and did not take medication overuse into account, found repressed hostility, sexuality issues, and unresolved dependency needs in patients with CTTH. The psychological problems these patients have could be the result, not the cause, of their chronic pain. Additionally, depression, anxiety, and chronic headache may be comorbid conditions with a common biological basis, as is true for the conditions of migraine, depression, and anxiety. Prior to the onset of either migraine or CTTH, patients show an increase in perceived stressful life events, whereas headache-free controls do not. This may be a result of an idiosyncratic, biologically determined overreaction to significant life events in these patients. Serotonin has been implicated in the genesis of migraine, depression, and anxiety disorders, and may be the biological basis for their comorbidity.

Treatment of tension-type headache

The approach to treating episodic headache, whether tension-type or migraine, is similar, and consists of psychophysiological therapy, physical therapy, and pharmacotherapy.

Psychophysiological therapy

Psychophysiological therapy involves reassurance, counselling, stress management, relaxation therapy, and biofeedback. (The use of traditional acupuncture is controversial and was not more effective than placebo in one study.) Although behavioural treatment of TTH may produce improvement more slowly than pharmacological treatment, improvement is often maintained for long periods without contact with the therapist. Relaxation and biofeedback are useful in the management of TTH. Relaxation training, EMG biofeedback training, or a combination of these can produce a 50% reduction in headache activity. This is a significantly greater decrease than observed in untreated patients or patients given placebo or sham biofeedback. Some patients who fail to respond to relaxation training may benefit from subsequent EMG biofeedback training.

Cognitive behavioural interventions, such as stress management programmes, may effectively reduce TTH activity when used alone, but these modalities may be more useful in conjunction with biofeedback or relaxation therapies, particularly in patients who have a high daily stress level. Biofeedback is especially helpful for patients who identify stress as a headache trigger and who are open to behavioural interventions. We often reserve biofeedback for patients who do not do well with relaxation exercises and tapes at home. When biofeedback is required, limited contact treatment utilizing three or four monthly clinical sessions supplemented by the home use of audiotapes and written materials is often a cost-effective alternative for many patients. Some patients require weekly treatment for several months to integrate the techniques. Excessive analgesic or ergotamine use limits the therapeutic benefits. Patients with continuous headaches are less responsive to relaxation or biofeedback therapies, and patients with significant psychiatric comorbidity may do poorly with behavioural treatment that does not address the comorbid problem. Younger patients and those who believe in nonconventional therapy often do well with biofeedback.

Physical therapy

Physical therapy consists of:

- modality treatments (heat, cold packs, ultrasound, and electrical stimulation);
- improvement of posture through stretching, exercise, and traction;
- trigger point injections or occipital nerve blocks; and
- a programme of regular exercise, stretching, balanced meals, and adequate sleep.

Physical therapy techniques include positioning, ergonomic instruction, massage, transcutaneous electrical nerve stimulation, hot or cold applications, and manipulations. While none of these techniques has proved effective in the long term, some (such as massage) may be useful for acute episodes of TTH.

Oromandibular treatment may be helpful for some TTH patients. Unfortunately, most studies that claim efficacy of such treatment as occlusal splints, therapeutic exercises for masticatory muscles, or occlusal adjustment are uncontrolled. Many headache-free subjects have signs and symptoms of oromandibular dysfunction; therefore, caution should be taken not to advocate irreversible dental treatments in TTH. In our experience, patients benefit infrequently from oromandibular treatment.

Pharmacotherapy

Pharmacotherapy consists of acute (abortive) therapy to stop or reduce the severity of the individual attack, using the following approaches:

- limited use of simple analgesics, alone or in combination with caffeine;
- limited use of either anxiolytics or codeine; and
- non-steroidal anti-inflammatory drugs (NSAIDs).

As a result of the potential for drug-induced headache, the use of these drugs must be limited (Table 7.2). Initiation of compound analgesics, anxiolytics, or codeine or other opiate agonists, alone or in combination, places a responsibility on the treating physician to arrange adequate

● **Table 7.2** *Acute medications for tension-type headache**

Drug		Efficacy	Side effects
Analgesics	Aspirin	2+	2
	Acetaminophen[†]	2+	1
Non-steroidal anti-inflammatory drugs	Indomethacin	3	2
	Ibuprofen	2+	2
	Naproxen	3+	2
	Fenoprofen	2	2
	Ketoprofen	2	2
	Ketorolac	3	3
Combination	Aspirin and/or acetaminophen[†] plus caffeine	3+	2
	Aspirin or acetaminophen[†] plus butalbital with caffeine	3+	3
Muscle relaxants	Orphenadrine	0 (?)	3
	Carisoprodol	0 (?)	3
	Methocarbamol	0 (?)	3
	Diazepam	0 (?)	3
	Cyclobenzaprine	0 (?)	3
	Chlorphenesin	0 (?)	3
	Chloroxazone	0 (?)	3

*Rated on a 1–3 scale.
[†]Paracetamol.

follow-up to assure that medication overuse does not develop.

Optimizing therapy requires knowledge of the range of treatments and awareness of the patient's preferences. Many acute treatments are available. The choice depends on the severity and frequency of the headaches, the associated symptoms, the presence of coexistent illness, and the patient's treatment profile. Oral medications, such as analgesics, NSAIDs, or a caffeine adjuvant compound are useful for patients with mild-to-moderate headaches that are not complicated by nausea. The simple guidelines are:

- use as simple a medicine as possible, such as paracetamol (acetaminophen), rather than an NSAID in the first instance;
- avoid combinations if possible, and particularly those with opiate agonists, such as codeine;
- avoid barbiturate use if possible; and
- as headaches become more difficult to

treat, ask the patient to complete a headache diary and be careful to arrange follow-up.

We begin with simple analgesics for patients with mild-to-moderate headaches. Many individuals find headache relief with over-the-counter (OTC) analgesics, such as paracetamol, aspirin, ibuprofen, naproxen, or ketoprofen. If these drugs fail, the addition of caffeine to aspirin and/or paracetamol has been demonstrated to provide pain relief. If OTC treatment is unsatisfactory, we use prescription drugs. The addition of butalbital, which is a barbiturate, to aspirin or paracetamol is helpful. The combination of paracetamol, isometheptene, and dichloralphenazone is also useful and more effective than simple analgesics, including NSAIDs, but great care must be used when prescribing butalbital-containing components because of the high potential for overuse. Avoid overuse of all analgesics because of the risk of dependence, abuse, and development of CDH.

Simple analgesics and NSAIDs are effective in TTH. Aspirin and paracetamol are more effective than placebo and are similar to each other. Ibuprofen, naproxen, and caffeine combinations are significantly more effective than placebo in controlled clinical trials. Ibuprofen (liquid) is more effective than paracetamol. Other NSAIDs, such as ketorolac or indomethacin, are also effective, but are less well studied. Based on the lower prevalence of gastrointestinal side effects, some doctors prefer ibuprofen and naproxen sodium.

The NSAIDs have anti-inflammatory, analgesic, and antipyretic properties and are quickly absorbed when taken orally, with a time to peak plasma concentration (T_{max}) of less than 2 hours. Naproxen has a plasma half-life of 14 hours, which accounts for its ability to provide pain relief that lasts 12 hours.

Some of the major side effects of NSAIDs include:

- gastrointestinal symptoms – epigastric discomfort, nausea, vomiting, gastritis, ulcers;
- dermatological symptoms – rash, pruritus;
- central nervous system side effects (less common) – headache, lethargy, confusion; and

- oedema, leucopenia, thrombocytopenia, liver-function abnormalities (rare).

Contraindications to NSAIDs include:

- hypersensitivity to aspirin or any NSAID;
- peptic ulcers;
- treatment with anticoagulants;
- bleeding tendency; and
- severe renal, cardiac, or liver impairment within the previous 3 months.

No evidence indicates that muscle relaxants, such as the mephenesin-like compounds, baclofen, diazepam, tizanidine, cyclobenzaprine, or dantrolene sodium, are effective in the treatment of TTH. However, the triptans are effective for TTH occurring in migraineurs.

Preventive treatment

Preventive treatment is designed to reduce the frequency and perhaps the severity of headache attacks and should be considered if the frequency (more than two attacks per week), duration (longer than 3–4 hours), or severity of attacks might lead to the overuse of abortive medication or significant disability. Preventive medication should also be considered if headache control is unsatisfactory after an adequate trial of non-pharmacological interventions and acute pharmacotherapy. If preventive medication is indicated, the agent should be chosen from one of the major categories, based on side-effect profiles and coexistent comorbid conditions (*see* Chapter 6).

Tricyclic antidepressants are the most widely used preventive agents for TTH, although controlled studies are sparse. Amitriptyline is the most frequently used tricyclic antidepressant. Other antidepressants, such as doxepin, nortriptyline, or protriptyline, can be used based on clinical experience. Selective serotonin reuptake inhibitors can also be used. They have fewer side effects than tricyclic antidepressants, and patients often prefer them. In one controlled trial, fluoxetine was more effective than placebo in a CDH group that included patients with CTTH.

Preventive drugs should be started at a low dose and increased slowly until therapeutic effects develop or the ceiling dose for the agent in question is reached. Tricyclic antidepressants, such as amitriptyline, are often used in doses of 75–200 mg/day for depression, while doses of 10–75 mg/day are often effective for TTH. With fluoxetine, for example, we begin with 10 mg and slowly increase the dose. Although some patients respond to lower doses of preventive medications, if the patient does not respond, the dose should be increased to tolerance before concluding that the agent is ineffective. A full therapeutic trial may take 2–6 months. Patients may be treated with a new preventive medication for 1–2 weeks without effect and then prematurely discontinue it, and both patient and physician believe it was not effective.

Judging the efficacy of a preventive medication can be difficult. Benefit may be limited if the patient is overusing analgesics. For this reason, the efficacy of preventive medications cannot be judged until medication overuse has been eliminated. Also, the benefit of treatment can be overestimated. Headaches may improve by coincidence independent of treatment or may remit after successful treatment; if headaches are well controlled for several months, preventive treatment should be tapered. Many patients experience continued relief after discontinuing medication; others may do well on a lower dose. Dose reduction may provide a better risk-to-benefit ratio. Other medications used to treat migraine and depression have also been used to treat ETTH and CTTH (*see* Chapter 6).

Summary

- TTH is the most common headache type.
- Headaches range from rare, brief episodes to frequent, often continuous, disabling headaches.
- No diagnostic tests exist for TTH, and therefore diagnosis requires exclusion of other organic disorders.
- Diagnosis is based chiefly on the absence of the characteristic symptoms of migraine.
- The physician must be alert to abnormalities on neurological examination, because secondary organic headache can mimic TTH.
- The pathogenesis of TTH may be similar to that of migraine – related to muscle tenderness, abnormal electromyogram and exteroceptive suppression of ES2, abnormal platelet serotonin, and decreased cerebrospinal fluid β-endorphin (in patients with severe CTTH).
- Treatment and prevention includes psychophysiological treatment, physical therapy, and pharmacotherapy.

Further reading

Iversen HK, Langemark M, Andersson PG, Hansen PE, Olesen J. Clinical characteristics of migraine and episodic tension-type headache in relation to old and new diagnostic criteria. *Headache* 1990; 30: 514–19.

Martin MJ, Rome HP, Swensom WM. Muscle contraction headache. A psychiatric review. *Res Clin Stud Headache* 1967; 1: 184–7.

Olesen J. Clinical and pathophysiological observations in migraine and tension-type headache explained by integration of vascular, supraspinal and myofascial inputs. *Pain* 1991; 46: 125–32.

Saper JR. Changing perspectives of chronic headache. *Clin J Pain* 1986; 2: 19–28.

Silberstein SD. Chronic daily headache and tension-type headache. *Neurology* 1993; 43:1644–9.

Silberstein SD, Lipton R, Solomon S, Mathew N. Classification of daily and near-daily headaches: proposed revisions to the IHS classification. *Headache* 1994; 34: 1–7.

Wittrock DA. The comparison of individuals with tension-type headache and headache-free controls on frontal EMG levels: a meta-analysis. *Headache* 1997; 37: 424–32.

8 Chronic daily headache: diagnosis and treatment

Introduction

Chronic daily headache (CDH) describes a heterogeneous group of headache disorders that occur more frequently than 15 days per month. Generally, CDH sufferers have headaches more days than not. Population-based studies in the United States and Europe suggest that 4–5% of the general population have CDH.

We classify CDH into two varieties, primary and secondary, and we subclassify the primary variety into headaches with an attack duration of less than 4 hours and headaches with an attack duration of more than 4 hours (Table 8.1). In this chapter, we describe some types of primary CDH that are not included in any part of the current International Headache Society (IHS) classifications – transformed migraine (TM), new daily persistent headache (NDPH), hemicrania continua, and hypnic headache. We concentrate on primary CDH with headache duration of more than 4 hours per discrete attack.

The lack of universal agreement about clinical groupings and diagnostic criteria for various types of CDH makes it difficult to classify patients. These diagnostic challenges have limited progress in developing new treatments. In addition, patients with CDH often overuse headache medication, which may initiate or sustain the pattern of frequent headaches, and thereby complicate diagnosis. Anxiety, depression, and other psychological disturbances often accompany CDH, complicate diagnosis, and require treatment.

Even in the absence of uniform terminology, physicians need a systematic approach to these difficult patients, in part to optimize treatment. We use the CDH rubric to start the classification process. For primary CDH disorders, if the headache duration is shorter than 4 hours per discrete attack, the differential diagnosis includes cluster headache, the paroxysmal hemicranias, idiopathic stabbing headache, hypnic headache, and other miscellaneous headache disorders. The differential diagnosis of these short-lasting CDHs is considered in Chapter 9. When the headache

● **Table 8.1** *Chronic daily headache*

Primary variety

Headache duration >4 hours
    Transformed migraine
    Chronic tension-type headache
    New daily persistent headache
    Hemicrania continua

Headache duration <4 hours
    Cluster headache
    Chronic paroxysmal hemicrania
    Hypnic headache
    Idiopathic stabbing headache

Secondary variety
Post-traumatic headache
Cervical spine disorders
Headache associated with vascular disorders: arteriovenous malformation; arteritis, including giant cell arteritis; dissection; subdural haematoma
Headache associated with non-vascular intracranial disorders (intracranial hypertension, infection [Epstein–Barr virus, human immunodeficiency virus], neoplasm)
Other (temporomandibular joint disorder; sinus infection)

duration is 4 hours or more, the major primary disorders to consider are chronic tension-type headache (CTTH), TM, hemicrania continua, and NDPH (Table 8.2). In the general population, CTTH constitutes 53.7% of CDH, while TM constitutes 31.7% of CDH. Although CTTH is more common, TM is more disabling.

Transformed migraine

Patients with TM usually have a history of episodic migraine, typically beginning in their teens or twenties. In headache clinics, most patients with TM are women, 90% of whom have a history of migraine without aura. The typical patient reports headaches that grow more frequent over months to years, while the associated symptoms of photophobia, phonophobia, and nausea become less severe and less prominent than in typical migraine. Patients often develop a pattern of daily or near daily headaches that resemble CTTH (i.e. the pain is

● **Table 8.2** *Headache classification for chronic daily headache*

Daily or near daily headache lasting >4 hours/day for >15 days/month

1.8 Transformed migraine

  1.8.1 with medication overuse

  1.8.2 without medication overuse

2.2 Chronic tension-type headache

  2.2.1 with medication overuse

  2.2.2 without medication overuse

4.7 New daily persistent headache

  4.7.1 with medication overuse

  4.7.2 without medication overuse

4.8 Hemicrania continua

  4.8.1 with medication overuse

  4.8.2 without medication overuse

Adapted from Silberstein et al., 1994

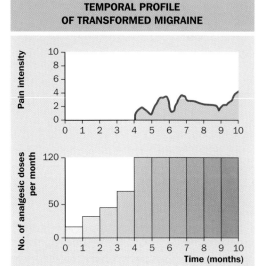

● **Figure 8.1** *Temporal profile of transformed migraine provided by a 30-year-old woman who has a 10 year history of headache. For many years she had bouts of episodic migraine without aura but with some nausea lasting 6–8 hours, which she treated with a caffeine–analgesic mixture. About 1 year previously her headaches became more frequent and she started to increase her use of analgesics. After 4 months she experienced daily, bilateral headaches which were mild to moderate in intensity and associated with periodic migraine exacerbations.*

often mild to moderate and not associated with photophobia, phonophobia, or gastrointestinal features). Other features of migraine, such as unilateral throbbing pain and aggravation by menstruation, or other migraine triggers, such as menstruation, may persist. In addition, attacks of full-blown migraine superimposed on a background of less severe headaches still occur in many patients.

In clinic-based samples, 80% of patients with TM overuse symptomatic medication. Headaches often increase in frequency when medication use increases (Figure 8.1). Stopping the overused medication usually results in an exacerbation, followed by distinct improvement, but often only after a delay of weeks or months (Figure 8.2). Many patients have significant long-term improvement after detoxification. In clinic-based samples, about 80% of patients with TM have depression, which often improves when the headaches improve and the medication overuse is interrupted.

Although TM is widely recognized as a clinical entity, formal diagnostic criteria are lacking. We believe that TM is a form of migraine and that diagnosis should ideally depend upon a past history of episodic IHS migraine with a pattern of headache acceleration (transformation). The period of transformation is characterized by increasing headache frequency and decreasing

prominence of associated migrainous features. Unfortunately, many patients with the characteristics and expected treatment–response profile of TM cannot recall the characteristics of prior headaches or the pattern of evolution. For these reasons, we proposed criteria that offer three alternative diagnostic links to migraine:

- prior history of migraine as defined by the IHS;
- clear period of escalating headache frequency with decreasing severity of migrainous features; and
- current superimposed attacks of headaches that meet all the IHS criteria for migraine with the exception of duration.

If all three features are present, then TM is clinically certain; if one or two features are present, we term this clinically probable TM.

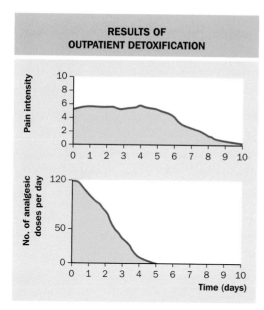

RESULTS OF OUTPATIENT DETOXIFICATION

● **Figure 8.2** *Results of outpatient detoxification. An improvement in CDH occurred within days of stopping the overuse of analgesics. Breakthrough headaches were treated with intramuscular dihydroergotamine administration. (Same patient as in Figure 8.1)*

Figure 8.2 illustrates the course of a patient with daily headache whose headache remitted, but whose episodic migraine continued when medication overuse was eliminated. In such a patient the diagnosis changes from episodic migraine to TM with medication overuse, then back to episodic migraine. Thus, it is important to limit the use of acute headache drugs. Although migraine transformation most often develops with medication overuse, it may also occur without overuse.

Other forms of chronic daily headache

Chronic tension-type headache

Also, CDH may develop in patients with a history of episodic tension-type headache (ETTH). These headaches are often diffuse or bilateral, frequently involving the posterior head and neck. In chronic tension-type headache (CTTH), in contrast to TM, most features of migraine are absent, as is prior or coexistent episodic migraine (Chapter 7).

New daily persistent headache

Occasionally, new daily persistent headache (NDPH) is seen in primary care and is often caused by a postviral syndrome. It is the abrupt development of a headache that does not remit, often in patients younger than those who have TM. Development of NDPH takes less than 3 days, and some patients remember the exact day or time the headache started. Although NDPH has characteristics that are similar to CTTH, no history of evolution from migraine or ETTH is found. However, classifying NDPH on the absence of a history of headache is difficult because almost 70% of men and 90% of women have had TTH at some time. Also, NDPH may be associated with medication overuse. It has some distinct causes, such as low cerebrospinal fluid pressure, and can be very difficult to treat. Referral to a neurologist or headache specialist is recommended for the evaluation of NDPH.

Hemicrania continua

Hemicrania continua, a headache disorder that occurs rarely, is characterized by a continuous, moderately severe, unilateral headache that varies in intensity and waxes and wanes without disappearing completely. The headache may alternate sides, although this is rare, and is frequently associated with jabs and jolts (idiopathic stabbing headache), as is migraine. Neck movements do not trigger hemicrania continua, but tender spots may be present. Exacerbations of pain are often associated with signs of autonomic disturbances on the side of the headache, such as ptosis, miosis, tearing, and sweating, as seen with cluster headache and related syndromes (*see* Chapter 9). Some patients may have photophobia, phonophobia, and nausea. Hemicrania continua almost always responds promptly to treatment with indomethacin. We have seen cases undiagnosed for decades. Many patients with hemicrania continua overuse acute medication, as do patients with most forms of primary CDH. Control of medication overuse often clarifies the underlying problem.

Many features of hemicrania continua resemble those of the short-lived trigeminal autonomic cephalalgias, such as chronic paroxysmal hemicrania, and both types respond to indomethacin. However, hemicrania continua is characterized by continuous moderate pain without autonomic features between the painful exacerbations, while the others have short-lived attacks with relative freedom from pain between attacks.

Drug overuse and rebound headache

Patients with frequent headache often overuse opioids, combination analgesics, ergotamine, and the triptans (Figure 8.3). Less commonly, simple analgesics may be overused. Medication overuse by headache-prone patients contributes to the development and maintenance of CDH (drug-induced rebound headache). In addition, medication overuse can make headaches refractory to preventive medication. When symptomatic medications are discontinued, headache exacerbation, as well as withdrawal symptoms (depending upon the overused medication), may occur. Headaches generally improve after that. After ergotamine or analgesics have been eliminated, many CDH patients stop having daily headaches, although episodic migraine attacks frequently continue. In headache clinics, most patients with drug-induced headache have a history of episodic migraine that has been converted into TM as a result of medication overuse. In headache clinics in the United States, as many as 50–80% of patients who present with CDH used analgesics on a daily or near-daily basis. In Europe, prevalence estimates of drug-induced headache vary by country, ranging from figures identical to the United States in the National Hospital in the United Kingdom to 5–10% in other centres.

With the exception of caffeine, analgesic rebound headache has not been demonstrated in placebo-controlled trials. Nonetheless, the existence of rebound headache is supported by clinical observation. Rebound headaches tend to occur at the end of dosing intervals as medication wears off. Headaches often occur in the early morning after overnight abstinence, or they may even awaken patients from sleep as the disorder progresses.

Medication overuse is defined quantitatively, based on the frequency and type of medication consumed. We consider overuse to be when patients take opioids or ergotamine tartrate more often than 2 days a week, three or more simple

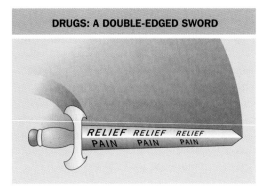

DRUGS: A DOUBLE-EDGED SWORD

RELIEF RELIEF RELIEF
PAIN PAIN PAIN

● *Figure 8.3* Overuse of medication by headache-prone patients frequently produces drug-induced CDH accompanied by dependence on symptomatic medication.

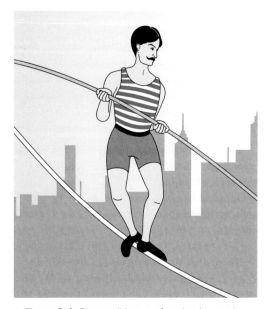

● *Figure 8.4* Responsible use of analgesics can be difficult!

analgesics a day for more than 5 days a week, or combination analgesics containing barbiturates, sedatives, or triptans for more than 3 days a week (Figure 8.4). To prevent rebound headache, we recommend specific limits for various acute drugs. The frequency of days of ergotamine use is as important, if not more important, than the total monthly dose. Rebound can develop in patients taking as little as 0.5–1.0 mg of ergotamine three times a week. Recent studies report that the triptans induce rebound

headache. We recommend limiting all the triptans (sumatriptan, naratriptan, rizatriptan, and
zolmitriptan) to 3 days a week and careful daily
monitoring by the physician when headache frequency is 2 days or more a week.

Most CDH patients overuse symptomatic medication, and some may develop psychological
dependence, tolerance, and abstinence syndromes. Medication overuse may be responsible
in part for the transformation of episodic migraine
or ETTH into daily headache and for the perpet-
uation of that syndrome. Medication overuse is
usually motivated by the patient's desire to treat
the headaches, and the desire of some patients to
treat their mood disturbance. While most CDH
patients overuse medication, others do not and
continue to have daily headaches long after the
overused medication has been discontinued.
While not all patients' headaches improve with
control of analgesic use, most feel better when
the overuse is controlled.

Other serious adverse effects of drug overuse
include:

- interference with preventive headache
  medications;
- renal or hepatic toxicity from large
  amounts of drug;
- tolerance (decreased effectiveness of the
  same dose, often leading to higher doses);
- habituation (psychological need to
  repeatedly use the drug); and
- dependence (physical need to repeatedly
  use the drug).

Psychiatric comorbidity

Anxiety, depression, and bipolar disease are more
frequent in migraine patients than in non-
migraine control subjects and probably in patients
with TM as well, since this disorder evolves from
migraine. Several headache clinics report that 80%
of patients with TM suffer from depression.
Clinical experience suggests that comorbid
depression often improves when the cycle of
daily head pain is broken. However, the biological relationship of migraine vulnerability to
rebound headache and psychiatric comorbidity
remains to be clarified.

Pathophysiology

The source of pain in CDH is unknown. Recent
studies suggest that it may result from one or
more of the following (*see* Chapter 5):

- abnormal excitation of peripheral nerves
  leading to pain perception with
  sensitization (an increase in reaction to a
  stimulus);
- enhanced responsiveness of the brainstem
  relay centre for head pain (the trigeminal
  cervical complex);
- defective pain modulation (the inability to
  turn off pain); and
- continuous activity of the brainstem areas
  associated with migraine.

Drug-induced headache mechanisms

The overuse of analgesics, barbiturates, opioids,
triptans, or ergots can contribute to the transformation of episodic headache into CDH. Some
investigators believe that drug-induced CDH
results from a rebound effect wherein medication
withdrawal triggers the next headache, which in
turn leads to increased drug consumption. This
may produce a vicious cycle that results in more
frequent drug use and drug-induced CDH. Drug
formulations that maintain sustained, non-fluctu-
ating levels might avoid the development of drug-
induced headache.

Drug overuse might be associated with relapse
for several reasons:

- loss of the therapeutic effect of the drug;
- rebound changes caused by drug
  withdrawal; or
- re-induction of the primary
  pathophysiological process with the
  occurrence of a new episode.

The transformation of episodic to chronic headache
or the development of new CDH probably results
from sensitization in the pathways of the trigeminal system. The response to painful stimulation
would become enhanced and non-painful stimuli
might be interpreted as painful. This could result

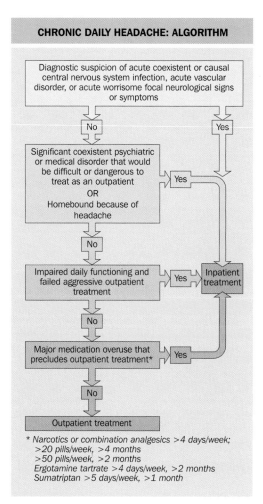

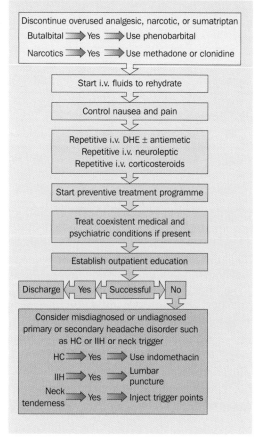

• **Figure 8.6** *CDH inpatient treatment algorithm. (DHE = dihydroergotamine; HC = hemicrania continua; IIH = idiopathic intracranial hypertension.)*

from neurochemical or hormonal changes, stressful events that could enhance pain perception, or an ongoing peripheral painful stimulus (because of other painful disorders in the trigeminal or cervical area). Chronic acute drug overuse could also alter the pain modulation system of the brainstem, resulting in central sensitization. Clinical strategies based on these concepts can be used in the long-term treatment of headache patients.

Treatment

Overview

Treating patients who have daily headache can be difficult (Figures 8.5–8.7), particularly if they

have overused medication or suffer comorbid depression. Effective management requires the following steps:

- exclude secondary headache disorders;
- diagnose the specific long-duration primary CDH disorder (i.e. TM, hemicrania continua, NDPH, or CTTH, described earlier in this chapter);
- identify comorbid medical and psychiatric conditions and treat appropriately;
- identify medication overuse and detoxify the patient by limiting all symptomatic medications, except possibly long-acting non-steroidal anti-inflammatory drugs

(NSAIDs; see detoxification section below);

- treat acute severe headache in the patient who has not overused symptomatic medication with strictly limited pharmacotherapy (see acute pharmacotherapy section below);
- start the patient on a programme of preventive medication based on the specific diagnosis (see preventive pharmacotherapy section below) to decrease reliance on symptomatic medication, explaining to the patient that the preventive drug may not become fully effective until medication overuse has been eliminated and the washout period completed;
- provide psychophysiological therapy as needed, including reassurance, counselling, stress management, relaxation therapy, and biofeedback (a study of acupuncture indicates that it is not more effective than placebo.);
- encourage regular exercise, stretching, balanced meals, and adequate sleep; and,
- provide physical therapy as needed, including:
  - modality treatments (such as heat, cold packs, ultrasound and electrical stimulation),
  - stretching, exercise, and traction,
  - trigger point injections (treating painful trigger areas in the neck may be particularly effective for intractable CDH);
  - occipital nerve blocks.

Acute pharmacotherapy

For patients who do not overuse symptomatic medication, acute severe headache can be treated with antimigraine drugs, including sumatriptan, eletriptan dihydroergotamine (DHE), zolmitriptan, naratriptan, rizatriptan, , and ergotamine, as well as opioids. These drugs must be severely limited to prevent rebound headaches that complicate treatment and require detoxification. The risk of rebound is much lower for DHE and the triptans than for analgesics, opioids, and ergotamine. Our experience indicates that rebound is extremely rare with DHE and uncommon with the triptans.

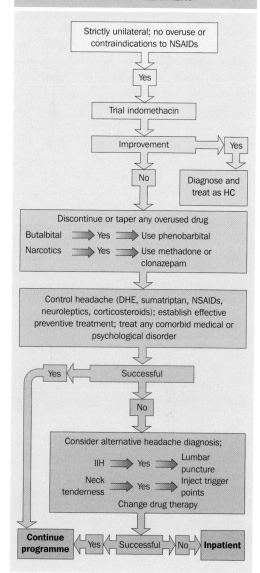

● **Figure 8.7** *CDH outpatient treatment algorithm. (NSAIDs = non-steroidal anti-inflammatory drugs; DHE = dihydroergotamine; HC = hemicrania continua; IIH = idiopathic intracranial hypertension.)*

Preventive pharmacotherapy

Patients with CDH should be treated primarily with preventive medications with the explicit understanding that medications may not become fully effective until overused medication has been eliminated and that it may take 3–6 weeks for treatment effect to develop.

The principles that guide the use of preventive treatment are:

- from among the first-line drugs, choose preventive agents based on their side-effect profiles, comorbid conditions, and specific indications (e.g. indomethacin for hemicrania continua);
- start at a low dose;
- gradually increase the dose until efficacy is achieved, until the patient develops side effects, or until the ceiling dose for the drug is reached;
- treatment effects develop over weeks, and treatment may not become fully effective until rebound is eliminated;
- if one drug fails, choose an alternative from another therapeutic class;
- prefer monotherapy, but be willing to use combination therapy; and
- communicate realistic expectations to the patient.

Most preventive agents used for CDH have not been examined in well-designed double-blind studies. Table 8.3 summarizes an assessment of the efficacy, safety, and evidence of a number of agents.

Antidepressants are attractive agents to treat CDH (TM, CTTH, and NDPH) since many patients have comorbid depression and anxiety. The most widely used are the tricyclic antidepressants, which include nortriptyline, amitriptyline, and doxepin. Start at 10–25 mg at bedtime and gradually increase the dose. Fluoxetine, a serotonin-specific reuptake inhibitor (SSRI), is coming into wider use for daily headaches, and evidence from a double-blind study demonstrates its efficacy in CDH. Fluvoxamine appears to be effective and may have analgesic properties. Other SSRIs, the new selective noradrenaline- (norepinephrine-) and serotonin-reuptake inhibitors, such as venlafaxine, and the monoamine oxidase inhibitors may have a therapeutic role, but this has not as yet been proved.

Beta-blockers (propranolol, nadolol), a mainstay of migraine therapy, are also used for CDH. Although clinicians fear that beta-blockers may exacerbate depression, this is unclear. As a result of the possibility of depression, beta-blockers are often used with antidepressants. Beta-blockers are

● **Table 8.3** *Summary of prophylactic drugs for use in chronic daily headache*

Drug	Clinical efficacy	Side effects	Clinical evidence[*]
Antidepressants			
Amitriptyline	+++	++	+++
Doxepin	+++	++	++
Fluoxetine	++	+	+++
Anticonvulsants			
Valproate	+++	++	++
Beta-blockers			
Propranolol, nadolol, etc.	++	+	+
Calcium-channel blockers			
Verapamil	++	+	+
Miscellaneous			
Methysergide	+++	+++	+

Modified from Tfelt-Hansen and Welch, 1993.
All categories are rated from + to ++++ based on a combination of published literature and clinical experience.
[*]Ratings of +++ for clinical evidence indicate at least one double-blind, placebo-controlled study. A rating of ++ indicates open well-designed studies and + indicates ratings based on clinical experience. A rating of ++++ requires at least two double-blind placebo-controlled trials.

relatively contraindicated in all patients with asthma, Raynaud's disease, and unstable diabetes.

Some, but not all, anticonvulsants are effective for migraine and CDH treatment. Sodium valproate (divalproex sodium) is an important drug for use in CDH, even in patients who have failed other agents. Four double-blind, placebo-controlled studies demonstrate sodium valproate's effectiveness in migraine, and smaller open studies demonstrate its efficacy in TM. Doses lower than those used for epilepsy (250 mg 2–3 times/day) may be sufficient, although we sometimes use up to 1200–1500 mg/day. Sodium valproate is an especially useful agent for patients with comorbid epilepsy and manic-depressive illness, and, possibly, anxiety disorders.

Open trials suggest that gabapentin may also be effective for CDH, but this needs to be more widely tested. The ergot derivative, methysergide, is an effective migraine preventive agent and is an option for CDH. It can be safely combined with tricyclic antidepressants, SSRIs, or calcium channel-blockers. The usual initial dose of methysergide is 2 mg twice a day, which can be increased to a maximum of 8 mg/day in four 2 mg doses; higher doses, although not recommended by the *Physicians' Desk Reference*, are sometimes useful.

The NSAIDs can be used for both symptomatic and preventive headache treatment and have been used for CDH. Naproxen sodium is effective for migraine prevention at a dose of one or two 275 mg tablets twice a day. Other NSAIDs include tolfenamic acid, ketoprofen, mefenamic acid, fenoprofen, and ibuprofen. Indomethacin is the drug of choice for hemicrania continua and chronic paroxysmal hemicrania, and the response to this medication contributes to the definition of these disorders. We give indomethacin a therapeutic trial (up to 150–225 mg/day for 1 week) to rule out hemicrania continua, but otherwise limit the use of other NSAIDs in patients with CDH.

Although monotherapy is preferred to avoid complex drug interactions and to increase compliance, it is sometimes necessary to combine preventive medications. Antidepressants are often used with beta-blockers or calcium channel-blockers, and sodium valproate may be used in combination with any of these medications.

Detoxification

Outpatient treatment, a preferred approach for motivated patients, is not always safe or effective and should be avoided when patients have significant coexistent medical diseases, such as coronary artery disease, epilepsy, labile hypertension, respiratory insufficiency, or renal or hepatic failure. However, it may be appropriate for patients who are overusing simple analgesics or NSAIDs and have no significant coexisting medical or psychiatric conditions. Inpatient detoxification is needed when patients have significant medical or psychiatric comorbidity, when outpatient detoxification is not safe, or when attempts to detoxify in an outpatient setting have failed. These patients are difficult to manage and often require referral to physicians with special expertise in headache disorders.

Outpatient

Two alternative strategies provide an approach to detoxifying the patient of overused medication in the outpatient setting:

- first start preventive therapy;
- then taper the overused medication, gradually substituting a long-acting NSAID; OR
- abruptly discontinue the overused drug, and either substitute an NSAID or use intramuscular DHE, neuroleptics, or corticosteroids (*see* Chapter 6 on migraine for details on dosage).

Serious withdrawal syndromes must be prevented. For example, if high doses of a butalbital-containing analgesic combination are abruptly discontinued, phenobarbital should be used to prevent barbiturate withdrawal. Similarly, benzodiazepines must be tapered.

Inpatient

Outpatient treatment is not always safe and frequently fails. If significant medical or psychiatric comorbidity is present, inpatient treatment is necessary. It is also needed if patients are overusing large amounts of butalbital-containing analgesics or opioids. The goals of inpatient treatment include:

- detoxification and rehydration;
- pain control with parenteral therapy (prochlorperazine, chlorpromazine, and DHE can be very useful);
- effective prophylaxis;
- patient education; and
- outpatient methods of pain control (i.e. give the patient the means to control headache without producing rebound).

Figure 8.8 illustrates a protocol that enhances and shortens detoxification and makes symptoms more tolerable to the patient. This protocol uses intravenous DHE with metoclopramide or domperidone to help control nausea. Following 10 mg of intravenous metoclopramide or a domperidone suppository, DHE 0.5 mg is administered intravenously. Subsequent doses are adjusted based on pain relief and side effects. Patients who are intolerant of DHE or who are not candidates for its administration (e.g. those with coronary artery disease or uncontrolled hypertension) may require repetitive intravenous neuroleptics (chlorpromazine, prochlorperazine, or droperidol) or corticosteroids, or both. These agents may also

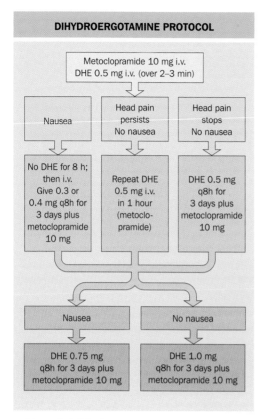

DIHYDROERGOTAMINE PROTOCOL

Metoclopramide 10 mg i.v.
DHE 0.5 mg i.v. (over 2–3 min)

Nausea

Head pain persists
No nausea

Head pain stops
No nausea

No DHE for 8 h; then i.v. Give 0.3 or 0.4 mg q8h for 3 days plus metoclopramide 10 mg

Repeat DHE 0.5 mg i.v. in 1 hour (metoclopramide)

DHE 0.5 mg q8h for 3 days plus metoclopramide 10 mg

Nausea

No nausea

DHE 0.75 mg q8h for 3 days plus metoclopramide 10 mg

DHE 1.0 mg q8h for 3 days plus metoclopramide 10 mg

● **Figure 8.8** *Dihydroergotamine treatment protocol. (After Raskin, 1986.)*

supplement repetitive intravenous DHE in refractory patients. Hospitalization is also used as a time for patient education, for introducing behavioural methods of pain control, such as biofeedback and relaxation techniques, and for adjusting an out-patient programme of preventive and acute therapy. In our experience, repetitive intravenous DHE is also a safe and effective means of rapidly controlling intractable headache.

Prognosis

For ethical and technical reasons, studying the natural history of CDH, particularly rebound headache, is difficult. Retrospective analysis suggests that patients may have periods of stable drug consumption and then accelerated drug use. In general, patients improve when they are treated aggressively. No studies report spontaneous improvement of rebound headache, although this may happen.

We did follow-up evaluations of 50 CDH patients who were hospitalized for drug overuse, treated with repetitive intravenous DHE, and became headache-free. Once detoxified, treated, and discharged, most patients did not resume daily analgesic or ergotamine use. At 3 months, 72% continued to show significant improvement, and 87% showed significant improvement after 2 years. Patients with drug-induced CDH, while difficult to treat, often return to a state of intermittent episodic headache after detoxification and treatment with a preventive medication. Our 2-year success rate of 87% is consistent with the long-term success rates reported in the literature.

Why treatment fails

When patients fail to respond to therapy or when they feel that they have tried everything and nothing works, treatment failure may be due to incomplete or incorrect diagnosis. For example:

- an undiagnosed secondary headache disorder may be the major source of the head pain, and the list in Table 8.4 should be considered;
- primary headache disorder may be misdiagnosed (i.e. hemicrania continua is mistaken for TM);
- two or more different headache disorders may be present;
- important exacerbating factors, such as medication overuse, may have been missed;
- pharmacotherapy may have been inadequate; or
- other factors may be present.

Prevention

Headache sufferers often do not realize that excessive or frequent self-treatment may perpetuate or exacerbate their headaches. Since most headache sufferers do not seek medical advice until the pain becomes frequent or intense, the opportunity for diagnosis and physician intervention to halt the overuse cycle is often missed. Therefore, physicians should specifically screen CDH patients for analgesic overuse and inform the patient about the risks of analgesic overuse and rebound headache. Yet, even when patients

● **Table 8.4** *Why treatment fails*

The diagnosis is incomplete or incorrect
An undiagnosed secondary headache disorder is present
A primary headache disorder is misdiagnosed
Two or more different headache disorders are present
Important exacerbating factors may have been missed
Medication overuse (including over-the-counter drugs)
Caffeine overuse
Dietary or lifestyle triggers
Hormonal triggers
Psychosocial factors
Other medications that trigger headaches
Pharmacotherapy has been inadequate
Ineffective drug
Excessive initial doses
Inadequate final doses
Inadequate duration of treatment
Other factors
Unrealistic expectations
Cormorbid conditions complicate therapy
Inpatient treatment required

are aware of the risks, they may still overmedicate, and this requires the physician's vigilance.

Patients who overuse medication may be unable to provide an accurate history of drug use. They often feel ashamed and out of control. The physician can explain the phenomenon of rebound headache and the importance of limiting doses of symptomatic headache medication (excepting possibly the long-acting NSAID).

Summary

- CDH refers to the broad group of headache disorders that occur more frequently than 15 days a month; this includes TM, CTTH, hemicrania continua, and NDPH.
- Patients with CDH are a diagnosis and treatment challenge because the clinical picture is often clouded by lack of an apparent structural or systemic cause, by therapeutic drug overuse, and by comorbidity.
- Patients frequently overuse their headache medication unaware that overuse causes rebound headache, dependence on symptomatic medication, and headache that is refractory to prophylactic medication.
- Effective management of CDH is best accomplished through accurate diagnosis, identifying comorbid conditions, detoxifying the patient from medication overuse, limiting pharmacotherapy and preventive medications, and patient education.
- Patients with CDH who are treated aggressively improve, and they sustain the improvement after detoxification and treatment with a preventive medication.
- Prevention of CDH includes the proper use of preventive medication and avoidance of drug overuse.

Further reading

Mathew NT, Kurman R, Perez F. Transformed or evolutive migraine. *Headache* 1987; 27: 102–6.

Newman LC, Lipton RB, Solomon S. Hemicrania continua: 7 new cases and a literature review. *Headache* 1993; 32: 237–8.

Newman LC, Lipton RB, Solomon S, Stewart WF. Daily headache in a population sample: results from the American Migraine Study. *Headache* 1994; 34: 295.

Raskin NH. Repetitive intravenous dihydroergotamine as therapy for intractable migraine. *Neurology* 1986; 36: 995–7.

Rasmussen BK. Migraine and tension-type headache in a general population: psychosocial factors. *Int J Epidemiol* 1992; 21: 1138–43.

Saper JR. Chronic headache syndrome. *Neurol Clin* 1989; 7: 387–412.

Physicians' Desk Reference. 53rd edition. Montoale NJ 1999

Scher AI, Stewart WF, Liberman J, Lipton RB. Prevalence of frequent headache in a population sample. *Headache* 1998; 38: 497–506.

Silberstein SD, Lipton RB. Chronic daily headache. In: Silberstein SD, Goadsby PJ (eds). *Blue Books of Practical Neurology: Headache*. Boston: Butterworth–Heinemann, 1997: 201–26.

Silberstein SD, Lipton RB, Goadsby PJ. Chronic daily headache. In: Silberstein SD, Lipton RB, Goadsby PJ (eds). *Headache in Clinical Practice*. Oxford: Isis Medical Media, 1998: 104–14.

Silberstein SD, Lipton RB, Sliwsinski M. Classification and daily and near-daily headaches: field trial of revised IHS criteria. *Neurology* 1996; 47: 871–5.

Tfelt-Hansen P, Welch KMA. Prioritizing prophylactic treatment. In: Olesen J, Tfelt Hansen P, Welch KMA (eds). *The Headaches*. New York: Raven Press Ltd, 1993: 403–5.

9 Cluster headache and related syndromes: diagnosis and treatment

Introduction

The general topic of this chapter is cluster headache, although its rare cousins that together form the trigeminal–autonomic cephalalgias (TACs) are included in the differential diagnosis for interest. As a group, the TACs generally have short attacks compared with migraine and are marked by prominent cranial autonomic symptoms, eye watering, or nasal stuffiness. The TACs, cluster headache, and related syndromes are among the most fascinating of the primary headaches; however, cluster headache itself is rare, and the related syndromes even more so. Including the rarer syndromes in a chapter that is predominantly about cluster headache is justified because a number of them can be treated effectively. Although similar in presentation, these headaches are treated differently. Interested readers are referred to the reading list at the end of this chapter for more complete coverage. At some point, a neurologist or headache specialist should be consulted to manage or advise about the patient with cluster headache and any of the related syndromes.

Patients with cluster headache present the image of a tortured sufferer, rocking or pacing in the dark, tears streaming from one eye, and face contorted in exquisite and devastating pain, with brief attacks occurring in a series that lasts for weeks or months. Chronic cluster headache can be a terrible problem that drives otherwise normal people to extraordinary acts. Cluster headache, which is a distinct, rare, clinical and epidemiological entity, is highly rewarding to manage. In the United Kingdom, cluster headache has been called 'migrainous neuralgia'. Other related short-lasting headaches with autonomic symptoms are less common, and these may be confused with cluster headache.

Clinical features

Once the physician determines that no intercurrent illness is present, the following International Headache Society criteria for cluster headache help to identify it:

- at least five attacks of severe, unilateral, orbital, suborbital, and/or temporal pain that last 15–180 minutes if untreated;
- at least one of conjunctival injection, lacrimation, nasal congestion, rhinorrhoea, forehead and facial sweating, miosis, ptosis, or eyelid oedema; and
- a typical frequency of one attack every other day to 6–8 attacks a day.

The features of cluster headache attacks are stereotypical. The attacks are generally shorter than those of migraine, lasting from 15–30 minutes to 2–3 hours, are almost always unilateral, and are located around the orbit or over the temporal regions. The level of pain, as reported by patients who have had other painful experiences, exceeds that of migraine, kidney stones, or childbirth. Attack frequency can range from one a day to two or more a day. Although eight attacks a day are said to be the maximum, this higher rate suggests other TACs. The significant features of cluster headache and other TACs are their clock-like regularity and cranial autonomic symptoms.

Differential diagnosis

Before the diagnosis of cluster headache can be made, other paroxysmal unilateral primary headache disorders and secondary headache disorders that mimic cluster headache must be excluded (Table 9.1). Most patients with the

● **Table 9.1** *Differential diagnosis of cluster headache*

Similar primary headaches	Similar secondary headaches	Secondary cluster headaches
Chronic paroxysmal hemicrania	Tolosa–Hunt syndrome	Meningioma of the lesser wing of sphenoid
Episodic paroxysmal hemicrania	Maxillary sinusitis	Vertebral artery dissection or aneurysm
SUNCT syndrome*	Temporal arteritis	High cervical meningioma
Hypnic headache	Raeder's paratrigeminal neuralgia	Head or neck injury
Cluster migraine		Pituitary adenoma
Trigeminal neuralgia		Occipital lobe atrioventricular malformation
		Facial trauma
		Orbito-sphenoidal aspergillosis
		Pseudoaneurysm of intracavernous carotid a.

*SUNCT = short-lasting unilateral neuralgiform headaches with conjunctival injection and tearing.

● **Table 9.2** *Differential diagnosis of primary short-lasting headaches*

Feature	Cluster headache	Chronic paroxysmal hemicrania	Episodic paroxysmal	SUNCT*	Idiopathic stabbing headache	Trigeminal neuralgia	Hemicrania continua	Hypnic Headache
Gender	M >F, 4:1	F > M, 3:1	F = M	M > F	F > M	F > M	F > M	F = M
Pain:								
type	Boring	Boring	Boring	Stabbing	Stabbing	Stabbing	Steady	Throbbing
severity	Very	Very	Very	Moderate	Severe	Very	Moderate	Moderate
location	Orbital	Orbital	Orbital	Orbital	Any	V2/V3>V1	Unilateral	bilateral (2/3)
Duration	15–180 min	2–45 min	1–30 min	15–240 s	≤1 s	<5 s	Continuous	15–30 min
Frequency	1–8/day	1–40/day	3–30/day	1/day to 30/h	Any	Any	Variable	1–3/night
Autonomic	+	+	+	+	−	−	+	−
Alcohol	+	−	−	−	−	−	−	−
Indomethacin	±	+	+	−	+	−	+	−

*SUNCT = short-lasting unilateral neuralgiform headaches with conjunctival injection and tearing.
V^1, ophthalmic; V^2, maxillary; V^3, mandibular divisions of the trigeminal nerve

typical syndrome show no organic cause, but a few patients have had lesions that were responsible for their headaches. Cluster-like headaches have also been reported among patients with arteriovenous malformation in the occipital lobe, pituitary adenoma, upper cervical meningioma, vertebral artery aneurysm, and dissection with ipsilateral pain. The differential diagnosis of the primary forms of short-lasting headache (Table 9.2) includes some very rare syndromes, such as paroxysmal hemicranias and hypnic headache. From a practical point of view, these syndromes should be considered if the patient's clinical picture is unusual. Atypical features include age greater than 55 years, female gender, very frequent attacks, or very short attacks. Patients who exhibit any of these characteristics should be referred to a neurologist or headache specialist (*see* Table 9.1).

Epidemiology

Epidemiological studies indicate that prevalence of cluster headache ranges between 0.09 and 0.4% of the population. Men are affected more frequently than are women (4.5–6.7:1.0), and the mean age of onset is 27–31 years.

Pathophysiology

The aetiology and pathophysiology of cluster headache is unknown. Some features overlap with those of other primary vascular headaches, such as migraine, and have a similar neurobiology. Pain around the eye implies involvement of the ophthalmic (first) division of the trigeminal nerve, and the autonomic symptoms of eye watering and blocked nose indicate parasympathetic involvement

(Figure 9.1). Historically, it has been held that the cavernous sinus may be a key locus of pathology, but recent positron emission tomography (PET) data establish that blood flow changes in that region are not limited to cluster headache. PET studies and special studies of brain structure using a new method called Voxel-based morphometry, indicate that the pathophysiology is driven partially or entirely from the central nervous system (Figure 9.2). The episodic nature of cluster headache, in which the headaches turn on and off like clockwork, seems to respect some daily (circadian) rhythm. Moreover, the remarkable half-yearly, yearly, or even biennial cycling of the bouts is one of the most fascinating cycling processes of human biology. The increase in attacks associated with the summer and winter solstice and the relative reduction of attacks around the equinoxes is remarkable. Cluster headache may be regarded as a dysfunction of neurons in the pacemaker or clock regions of the brain (posterior hypothalamus) that allows activation of a trigeminal–autonomic loop in the brainstem (Figure 9.3).

Treatment

Pharmacological treatment for cluster headache can be abortive (acute; Table 9.3), prophylactic (preventive; Table 9.4), or a combination of both. Abortive treatment is directed at managing the individual attack. Preventive treatment is directed at shortening the bouts of episodic cluster and controlling the frequency of attacks in both the episodic and chronic forms of the disorder. The physician can offer general advice about avoiding triggers, such as alcohol, nitrates, or organic solvents (paint thinner).

Management of acute attacks

Since cluster headache is rare, it seems appropriate for all diagnosed patients to be referred to a neurologist or headache specialist for evaluation. This is not to discourage their management by primary care doctors, but to recognize that this condition is uncommon and sometimes difficult to manage.

Treatments for the sudden-onset, short-duration, acute attacks of cluster headache include oxygen inhalation, sumatriptan, ergotamine, dihydroergotamine (DHE), and local anaesthetics

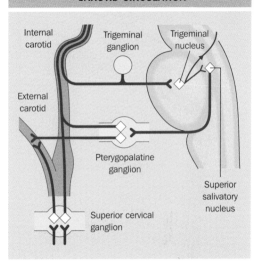

NEURAL INNERVATION OF THE CAROTID CIRCULATION

Internal carotid
Trigeminal ganglion
Trigeminal nucleus
External carotid
Pterygopalatine ganglion
Superior salivatory nucleus
Superior cervical ganglion

● **Figure 9.1** *The neural innervation of the carotid circulation and its relevance to cluster headache are illustrated. Sympathetic fibres arise in the superior cervical ganglion and follow the external and internal carotid arteries, while the parasympathetic innervation arises from neurons in the superior salivatory nucleus of the pons and projects mainly via the pterygopalatine ganglion. A reflex connection between the trigeminal innervation via the trigeminal ganglion activates these parasympathetic neurons with carotid dilation, leading to a compressive lesion of the sympathetic nerves, and thus pain, parasympathetic activation (red, watering eye and blocked nose), and sympathetic dysfunction (ptosis and pupillary change), characterize attacks of cluster headache.*

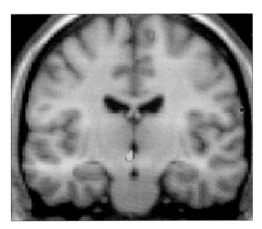

● **Figure 9.2** *Positron emission tomography scan demonstrating activation in the posterior hypothalamic grey matter in acute cluster headache. (Reproduced from May et al., 1998.)*

PATHOGENESIS OF CLUSTER HEADACHE

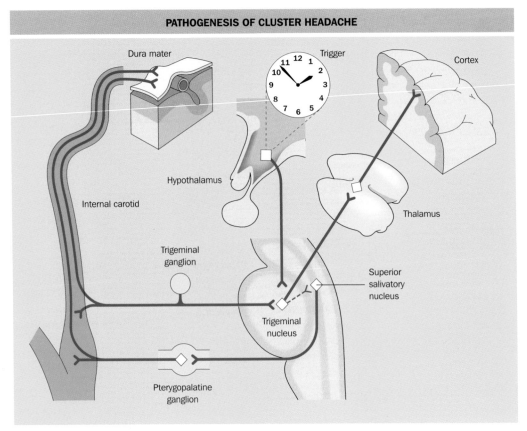

● **Figure 9.3** *An integrated model for cluster headache. The clock-regions of the hypothalamic grey (Figure 9.2) are active and involved in dysfunction of* the trigeminal–autonomic reflex (Figure 9.1), which leads to pain with autonomic features in the pattern of cluster headache.

● **Table 9.3** *Treatment of acute cluster headache*

- 100% oxygen at 10 l/min for 15 minutes
- Sumatriptan 6 mg subcutaneously
- Dihydroergotamine 1 mg intramuscularly or intravenously
- Lidocaine (lignocaine) 4–6% 2–3 times intranasally to the affected side

● **Table 9.4** *Prophylactic or preventive treatment of cluster headache*

Episodic cluster headache	Chronic cluster headache
Verapamil	Verapamil
Methysergide	Lithium carbonate
Corticosteroids	Valproate
Ergotamine	Methysergide
Valproate	

(Table 9.3). The short latency to the peak of pain makes parenteral or pulmonary drug administration highly beneficial. Oxygen inhalation, subcutaneous sumatriptan, and DHE by injection afford the fastest relief. Local intranasal anaesthetic agents (cocaine, lignocaine [lidocaine]) have occasionally been effective. Most ergotamine preparations, with the exception of parenteral DHE or ergotamine by inhalation, are too slowly absorbed to be effective in the acute attack.

Oxygen

Oxygen inhalation, a standard abortive treatment for cluster headache, is given via a non-rebreathing mask at a flow rate of 10 l/min for 15 minutes and can be safely used for repeated attacks. This is effective in approximately 70% of patients, usually within 10 minutes. In some patients, oxygen may delay rather than abort the attack, and pain may return. Oxygen's effectiveness may depend on the timing of administration – it may be most effective when given at the maximum intensity of the pain. High flow, high oxygen percentage, and a reasonable time period of inhalation are all key elements in treatment success. Several studies have also reported benefit from hyperbaric oxygen, but no more so than from normobaric oxygen, which is much more practical.

Sumatriptan

The 5-hydroxytryptamine 1B/1D (5-HT$_{1B/1D}$) agonist, sumatriptan, given as a 6 mg subcutaneous injection for a maximum of two attacks in 24 hours, works rapidly and efficiently, often producing benefit within 5–7 minutes of administration. Sumatriptan is contraindicated for patients with ischaemic heart disease, uncontrolled hypertension, and cerebrovascular disease. The mechanisms of action of sumatriptan in cluster headache are likely to be similar to those described in migraine (*see* Chapter 5), and the peripheral and central sites of action of the class are illustrated in Figure 5.12.

Dihydroergotamine

Acute attacks of cluster headache are relieved effectively by DHE. Intravenous injection gives more rapid relief than intramuscular injection, with benefit in less than 10 minutes. In some countries DHE nasal spray is also available. In a double-blind comparative trial of DHE nasal spray (1 mg; half the recommended dose for migraine), DHE did not change the duration or frequency of the attacks, but it did decrease pain intensity. Since DHE as a nasal spray has a 40% bioavailability, administration of a higher dose may be more effective for the treatment of cluster headache.

Ergotamine

Ergotamine tartrate (available as a tablet, suppository, or, in some countries, as an inhalant) may only partially ameliorate an acute cluster attack because of the preparation's pharmacokinetics. Some patients may respond to rectal ergotamine.

Topical local anaesthetics

Local intranasal anaesthetic agents, such as lignocaine (lidocaine), have been reported effective. Lignocaine 4–6% nasal drops (1 ml) may be used and repeated once after 15 minutes.

Analgesics and narcotics

Non-parenteral analgesics and narcotics have little role in treating cluster headache, although cluster headache patients are generally less susceptible to analgesic overuse problems. Such treatment would certainly require specialist monitoring.

Prophylactic pharmacotherapy of cluster headache

Preventive treatment in cluster headache is aimed at shortening bouts and controlling attack frequency. Although all the treatments are largely empirical, many are very effective. Most cluster patients require prophylactic therapy at some point because:

- attacks are frequent, severe, of rapid onset, and often too short-lived for abortive medication to take effect;
- abortive treatment may only postpone the attack;
- treating frequent attacks with abortive medications may result in overmedication; and
- failing to stop the cluster period early may prolong the suffering for months.

Medications effective in prophylactic treatment of cluster headache are listed in Table 9.4. Chlorpromazine, β-blockers, antidepressants, and histamine desensitization are probably ineffective as prophylaxis. Corticosteroids are not recommended for the treatment of chronic cluster because of the long-term effects. The goal is rapid remission of headache and maintaining that remission with minimal side effects until the cluster period is over. Recent open studies suggest that gabapentin and topiramate may be useful in cluster headache, but these require further study and must be regarded as a specialist initiative.

The principles of prophylactic pharmacotherapy are:

- start medications early in the cluster period;
- continue the drugs until the patient is headache-free for at least 2 weeks;
- taper the drugs rather then abruptly withdrawing them; and
- restart the drugs at the beginning of the next cluster period.

If an acute attack occurs despite preventive treatment, abortive agents as listed in Table 9.3 can be used.

The medication choice depends on:

- previous drug response;
- prior adverse drug reactions;
- contraindications to drug use;
- type of cluster (episodic or chronic);
- frequency and timing of attacks (nocturnal versus diurnal);
- expected length of cluster period; and
- age and lifestyle of the patient.

Combinations of two or more drugs may be necessary.

Ergotamine

Like DHE, ergotamine tartrate is an agonist at 5-$HT_{1B/1D}$ receptors, as is sumatriptan, and shares many of its pre-clinical actions (*see* Chapter 5). Ergotamine tartrate, up to 4 mg (in divided doses), is effective and probably poses no risk of rebound headache, unlike its use for migraine. Ergotamine is particularly useful in controlling nocturnal attacks when taken at bedtime.

Methysergide maleate

Methysergide maleate is a congener of methylergonovine and lysergic acid diethylamide that is widely distributed throughout the body, crosses the blood–brain barrier, and binds to serotonin receptors in the brain. It has affinity for 5-HT_1 and 5-HT_2 receptors, but its mechanism of action is unclear. Methysergide is effective in 65–69% of patients with episodic cluster headache, but response rates are lower in chronic cluster. This drug is indicated in younger patients, who do not have the potential risk of atherosclerotic heart disease. Side effects include muscle cramps, nausea, diarrhoea, and abdominal discomfort; these often occur initially, but usually subside over several days. Prolonged treatment has been associated with fibrotic reactions (retroperitoneal, pleural, pulmonary, and cardiac valvular), although these are rare. Since the duration of episodic cluster headache is less than 4 months, methysergide use in general does not cause this complication. In chronic cluster headache, however, methysergide has to be used with caution to include a 1-month drug holiday

between 6-month treatment periods. If methysergide use is prolonged and a drug holiday is omitted, renal function studies periodic chest radiography, echocardiogram, and magnetic resonance imaging of the abdomen must be performed.

Calcium-channel blockers – verapamil

Verapamil has been studied in the treatment of cluster headache, and many physicians, including the authors, believe it is the prophylactic drug of choice in some patients with episodic and most patients with chronic cluster headache. Doses range between 120 and 600 mg *daily*, but much higher doses up to 720 mg *daily* have been used safely. Such high doses require specialist supervision and careful monitoring of cardiac status, being particularly alert for AV node conduction problems. Constipation is the most common side effect. Other symptoms include oedema, dizziness, nausea, hypotension, and fatigue. Verapamil can be combined with ergotamine or lithium. When verapamil and lithium are used together, sensitivity to lithium may be increased. In one double-blind trial, verapamil was found to be as effective as lithium.

Lithium carbonate

Lithium's mode of action in cluster headache (and in manic-depressive illness) is unknown. It alters circadian rhythms and diminishes rapid eye movement in sleep. Lithium is more effective in chronic than in episodic cluster headache. The response of patients with chronic cluster headache is 78% and that of patients with episodic cluster headache is 63%. The usual initial dose of lithium is 300 mg twice daily, but higher doses may be required. Lithium has a long half-life (24 hours) and takes about 1 week to reach steady-state levels, at which time the lithium level should be obtained (and periodically thereafter). Lithium is often effective at a blood level of 0.4–0.8 mmol/l, which is less than the usual dose for mania. A therapeutic response is often seen within 1 week. Approximately 20% of chronic cluster headache may become episodic on lithium treatment, and many patients require an additional agent, such as ergotamine or verapamil, along with lithium. Some patients eventually become resistant to lithium.

Side effects of lithium include slight weakness, mild nausea, and thirst, which usually subside, tremor, lethargy, slurred speech, and blurred vision. Toxicity is manifested by nausea, vomiting, anorexia, diarrhoea, and neurological signs of confusion, nystagmus, ataxia, extrapyramidal signs, and seizures. Concomitant use of sodium-depleting diuretics should be avoided, as sodium depletion results in high lithium levels and neurotoxicity. An interaction with indomethacin to increase lithium levels should be noted in the context of indomethacin-sensitive headaches (*see* Table 9.2). Hypothyroidism and polyuria (nephrogenic diabetes insipidus) can occur with long-term use. Polymorphonuclear leukocytosis can occur and be mistaken for occult infection.

Corticosteroids

The mechanism of action of corticosteroids in cluster headache is uncertain. Corticosteroids (prednisone and dexamethasone) are the most rapid-acting of the prophylactic drugs used in the treatment of cluster headache and are frequently used short-term (2–3 weeks in tapering doses) as initial therapy to induce remission. This may break the headache cycle while waiting for other drugs to become effective. Prednisone produced relief in 77% of cluster headache patients, partial improvement in 12%, and total relief in up to 50%. Dexamethasone (4 mg twice daily for 2 weeks, 4 mg/day for 1 week) is also effective. Corticosteroids are also useful in chronic cluster headache; however, as in episodic cluster, when the medication is tapered, the headache recurs. Since the side effects of corticosteroids increase with long-term use, their use is limited to inducing remission and in occasional patients with refractory chronic cluster to provide a holiday from their attacks. Adverse effects include insomnia, restlessness, personality changes, hyponatraemia, oedema, hyperglycaemia, osteoporosis, myopathy, and gastric ulcers. Recently, necrosis of the hip has been reported, and this is an important side effect to consider and warn patients about.

Sodium valproate

Sodium valproate (divalproex sodium), 250–2000 mg/day, given usually as a divided dose twice daily, has been reported to be effective in cluster headache. Treatment was well tolerated with only nausea reported. Lethargy, weight gain, tremor and hair loss are some of the common side effects. With valproate use, pancreatitis and liver function abnormalities are rarer but more severe adverse events. The valproate level should be maintained between 50 and 120 mg/ml (400–600 µmol/l). Liver-function studies and blood counts should be obtained prior to initiating treatment and during follow-up if the patient is symptomatic. Valproate should not be used for patients with liver disease.

Capsaicin

Capsaicin desensitizes sensory neurons by depleting substance P. In a double-blind, placebo-controlled study using capsaicin (0.025% cream twice daily) applied intranasally via a cotton-tipped applicator on the side of headache for 7 days, patients who received the active drug had significantly less frequent and less severe attacks. The application is very unpleasant.

Indomethacin

Indomethacin is particularly useful in treating both chronic and episodic paroxysmal hemicrania, and although some cluster headache patients have fewer headaches when taking it, the significance of this response is unknown (*see* Table 9.2). While the response to indomethacin is absolute in paroxysmal hemicrania and hemicrania continua, it is only partial in the other entities, including cluster headache.

Some treatment protocols

Many clinicians start treatment of episodic cluster headache with verapamil 120–480 mg/day. Other clinicians start with ergotamine tartrate 1–4 mg/day, particularly for patients with nocturnal attacks, in which a dose is given at bedtime, although this precludes use of sumatriptan. Ergotamine can be used alone or in combination with verapamil. Methysergide 1–2 mg taken 3–4 times a day is an effective alternative, especially for younger patients. Methysergide should not be combined with ergotamine. Lithium or valproate can be used next, alone or in combination with verapamil. Corticosteroids may be used to break the cycle of headache or to treat severe exacerbations. Pizotifen is recommended by some physicians for cluster headache, but we have not found it useful.

Chronic cluster headache can be treated with verapamil or lithium, alone or in combination. In resistant cases, triple therapy using either ergotamine, verapamil, and lithium or methysergide, verapamil, and lithium may be considered. Valproate can be used alone or in combination with verapamil or methysergide. Patients who are difficult to manage need regular specialist review.

In studies of sumatriptan as a preventive in cluster headache, the drug was administered at a dose of 100 mg three times daily, and no change in the frequency of attacks was observed over the placebo. Acetazolamide may be a useful pre-treatment for patients whose attacks are triggered by altitude, such as a ski trip. Kudrow (1980) suggests 250 mg twice daily for 4 days commencing 2 days prior to going to a high altitude.

The treatment-resistant patient and options for surgical procedures

The patient with episodic cluster may become resistant to a previously successful prophylactic medication. The chronic cluster patient may require polypharmacy and eventually an ablative neurosurgical procedure. For the patient with cluster headache that is resistant to treatment, the primary care physician should consider referral to a neurologist, particularly one who specializes in headache.

Patients may be candidates for surgical consideration for the following indications:

- strictly unilateral headache;
- total resistance to medical therapy or significant contraindications to effective medical therapy; and
- a stable personality profile with no addictive potential.

The procedure of choice is radiofrequency thermocoagulation of the trigeminal ganglion. The overall results have been encouraging, with almost 75% of patients becoming free of cluster headache attacks.

Summary

- Cluster headache is a relatively rare type of headache characterized by excruciating pain and autonomic symptoms that occur for short periods in a series.
- The aetiology and pathophysiology of cluster headache is not yet fully understood, but the pattern of pain and the pattern of the episodes suggest central nervous system dysfunction, and PET studies identify the region of the posterior hypothalamic grey matter as being pivotal in the process.
- Like migraine, pharmacological treatment for cluster headache is abortive or preventive, or both.
- Patients with total resistance to medical therapy or who have contraindications to effective medical therapy may be candidates for surgical procedure, usually radiofrequency thermocoagulation of the trigeminal ganglion.

Further reading

Goadsby PJ, Lipton RB. A review of paroxysmal hemicranias, SUNCT syndrome and other short-lasting headaches with autonomic features, including new cases. *Brain* 1997; 120: 193–209.

Lance JW, Goadsby PJ. *Mechanism and Management of Headache*. London: Butterworth–Heinemann, 1998.

Kudrow L. *Cluster Headache: Mechanisms and Management*. Oxford: Oxford University Press, 1980.

May A, Bahra A, Buchel C, Frackowiak RSJ, Goadsby PJ. Hypothalamic activation in cluster headache attacks. *The Lancet* 1998; 351: 275–8.

May A, Ashburner J, Buchel C, McGonigle DJ, Frackowiak RSJ, Goadsby PJ, Correlation between structural and functional changes in brain in an idiopathic headache syndrome. *Nature Med* 1999; 5: 836–38.

Silberstein SD, Lipton RB, Goadsby PJ. *Headache in Clinical Practice*. Oxford: ISIS Medical Media, 1998.

Sjaastad O. *Cluster Headache Syndrome*. London: WB Saunders, 1992.

Secondary headache disorders

10 Post-traumatic headache

Introduction

Post-traumatic headache (PTH) is a secondary headache that arises after head injury and is often part of the post-traumatic syndrome. It usually follows mild-to-moderate closed head injury even without loss of consciousness. In addition to headache, symptoms include depression, irritability, memory impairment, loss of libido, dizziness or vertigo, alcohol intolerance, and attention and concentration difficulties. Most physicians agree that some patients develop PTH as a sequela to cranial injury, but this relationship is unclear. Medicolegal complications interfere with patient care and cast doubt on the existence of this disorder; however, in countries that do not have litigation problems, the prevalence and disability from PTH are the same as they are in countries that do. In this chapter, we discuss the epidemiology, diagnosis, pathophysiology, diagnostic testing, and management of patients with PTH.

Epidemiology

Head injuries have three major causes – motor vehicle accidents (which account for 45% of head injuries), falls (which account for 30%), and occupational and recreational accidents (20%). Each year, approximately 200/100,000 individuals with mild head injury (defined as a Glasgow coma scale of 13–15; Table 10.1) are hospitalized. Many of these patients develop PTH. Whiplash refers to the extension, flexion, and lateral motions of the neck that follow impact, with or without direct trauma to the head. Whiplash injuries are followed by symptoms that resemble the post-traumatic syndrome and include neck pain, headaches, dizziness, and paraesthesias. Cognitive and psychological sequelae are extremely common in both PTH and whiplash.

Clinical features

The International Headache Society (IHS) defines PTH based on the temporal relationship of the headache to the trauma, not on the headache's symptom profile. The criteria require headache onset to occur within 2 weeks of head injury or, if consciousness is lost, upon regaining consciousness (Table 10.2). However, in clinical practice the onset of PTH may be obscured by pain caused by direct injury to the head, face, or neck, which makes the IHS criteria difficult to apply.

Special types of PTH

Trauma may exacerbate a pre-existing primary headache disorder, such as migraine, cluster, or tension-type headache. It may also be an initiating event, producing the first of many headache attacks. The essence of the diagnosis is that cranial trauma initiated the headache, which is often associated with symptoms of post-traumatic syndrome, such as vertigo, blurred vision, and cognitive complaints. Post-traumatic syndrome symptoms (Table 10.3) may either be delayed or develop immediately following the trauma.

Impaired memory and difficulty concentrating are common in post-traumatic syndrome. Some patients have neurocognitive deficits, including anger, depression, irritability, personality change, and inability to process information (making them appear absent-minded). Also, PTH is associated with non-specific episodic or positional dizziness. Sleep disturbances, such as insomnia and daytime drowsiness, are frequent. Dizziness and periodic loss of consciousness are rare.

● **Table 10.1** *Glasgow coma scale*

Eye opening (E)		Best motor response (M)	
Spontaneous	4	Obeys	6
To sound	3	Localizes	5
To pain	2	Withdraws	4
None	1	Abnormal flexion	3
Verbal response (V)		Extends	2
		None	1
Oriented	5		
Confused	4		
Inappropriate	3		
Incomprehensible	2	Score = E + M + V, and	
None	1	ranges between 3 and 15	

● **Table 10.2** *IHS criteria for post-traumatic headache*

5.1 Acute post-traumatic headache

5.1.1 With significant head trauma and/or confirmatory signs

Diagnostic criteria:

A Significance of head trauma documented by at least one of the following:

   1 Loss of consciousness

   2 Post-traumatic amnesia lasting more than 10 minutes

   3 At least two of the following exhibit relevant abnormality: clinical neurological examination, radiography of the skull, neuroimaging, evoked potentials, spinal fluid examination, vestibular function test, neuropsychological testing

B Headache occurs less than 14 days after regaining consciousness (or after the trauma, if there has been no loss of consciousness)

C Headache disappears within 8 weeks after regaining consciousness (or after trauma, if there has been no loss of consciousness)

5.1.2 With minor head trauma and no confirmatory signs

Diagnostic criteria:

A Head trauma that does not satisfy 5.1.1A

B Headache occurs less than 14 days after injury

C Headache disappears within 8 weeks after injury

5.2 Chronic post-traumatic headache

A Significance of head trauma documented by at least one of the following:

   1 Loss of consciousness

   2 Post-traumatic amnesia lasting more than 10 minutes

   3 At least two of the following exhibit relevant abnormality: clinical neurological examination, radiography of the skull, neuroimaging, evoked potentials, spinal fluid examination, vestibular function test, neuropsychological testing

B Headache occurs less than 14 days after regaining consciousness (or after the trauma, if there has been no loss of consciousness)

C Headache continues for more than 8 weeks after regainingconsciousness (or after trauma, if there has been no loss of consciousness)

5.2.2 With minor head trauma and no confirmatory signs

Diagnostic criteria:

A Head trauma that does not satisfy 5.1.1A

B Headache occurs less than 14 days after injury

C Headache continues for more than 8 weeks after injury

After Headache Classification Committee of the International Headache Society, 1988.

● **Table 10.3** *Sequelae of mild head injury*

Headaches	Psychological and somatic complaints
Tension-type	Irritability
Migraine	Anxiety
Cluster	Depression
Low cerebrospinal pressure	Personality change
Occipital neuralgia	Fatigue
Idiopathic intracranial hypotension	Sleep disturbance
Supraorbital and infraorbital neuralgia	Decreased libido
	Decreased appetite
Cervicogenic	**Rare sequelae**
Temporomandibular joint syndrome or dysfunction	Subdural and epidural haematomas
Local neuroma	Seizures
Mixed	Transient global amnesia
Cranial nerve symptoms and signs	Tremor
	Dystonia
Dizziness	
Vertigo	
Tinnitus	
Hearing loss	
Blurred vision	
Diplopia	
Convergence insufficiency	
Light and noise sensitivity	
Diminished taste and smell	

Following head injury, orthostatic headache (a headache that occurs with standing and is relieved with recumbency) can occur because of a cerebrospinal fluid (CSF) leak through a dural root sleeve tear or a cribriform plate fracture, among other causes. These headaches, like post-lumbar puncture headaches, are a consequence of intracranial hypotension and have similar clinical features. Temporomandibular joint injury may occur, with symptoms of incomplete jaw opening, clicking, jaw pain with chewing, and pain on palpation of the jaw joint or the muscles of mastication. Temporomandibular joint dysfunction may be a headache trigger.

Risk factors

Age, gender, and certain mechanical factors are risks for a poor outcome after a head injury or whiplash injury. Women have twice the risk of PTH compared with men. Older patients have a slower and less complete recovery. If the head is inclined or rotated at impact in a vehicle collision, of if the collision is rear-end or an occupant is unprepared, PTH is more likely to result. The relationship between the severity of the injury and the severity or incidence of PTH is uncertain. Headache persistence does not correlate with the presence of post-traumatic amnesia, skull fracture, electroencephalogram abnormalities, bloody CSF, or the duration of unconsciousness.

Pathophysiology

As a group, PTHs are trauma-induced disorders with overlapping symptoms. Peripheral nerve injury may result in burning or lancinating neuralgic pain; soft-tissue or skeletal injuries may initiate or trigger chronic daily headache; and injury to the neck, jaw, and tissues of the scalp may cause pain that is referred into the head. Any head trauma, not necessarily direct impact, that causes shear forces to the brain can produce axonal injury, most commonly to the corpus callosum, internal capsule, fornices, dorsolateral midbrain, and pons. Head injury usually involves translational and rotational forces. This results in the different parts of the brain, such as the cerebral hemispheres and the cerebellum, moving out of synchrony, which makes axons in the upper brainstem particularly vulnerable to diffuse axonal injury. Midbrain haemorrhage can result, and ischaemic brain injury, abnormal cerebrovascular autoregulation, and vasospasm may follow severe headache (Figure 10.1).

Testing

Anatomic imaging

Most patients who require hospitalization as a result of mild or moderate head injury have magnetic resonance imaging (MRI) abnormalities, which often spontaneously resolve within 1 month. All acute PTH patients should have neuroimaging if they exhibit:

- Glasgow coma scale lower than 15;
- mild behavioural abnormalities; or
- any equivocal findings on examination.

When patients present several weeks after injury with subacute or chronic post-traumatic syndrome,

BRAIN MOTION

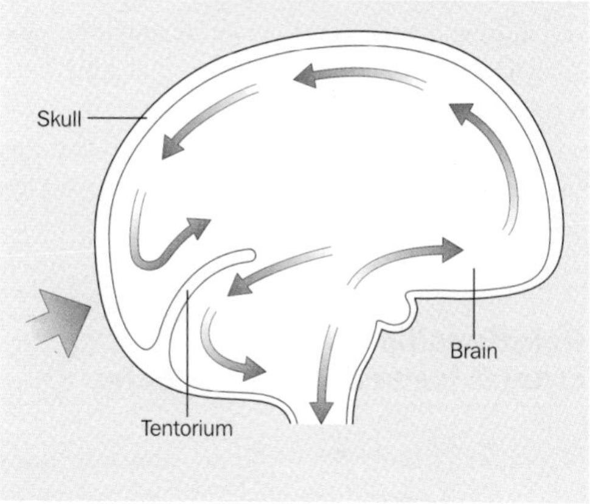

● **Figure 10.1** Brain motion. (Adapted with permission from Ward, 1981.)

the guidelines for neuroimaging are less clear. If headaches persist and neuroimaging was not carried out following the injury, brain CT or MRI should be performed to exclude chronic subdural haematoma, hydrocephalus, or a structural lesion unrelated to the trauma. Prominent and persistent neck pain is an indication for a cervical MRI, but if the neurological examination is normal or severe radicular symptoms are absent, an abnormal MRI does not change therapy. If fracture or dislocation of the cervical spine is suspected, it must be ruled out by radiography.

Physiological testing

Electroencephalography is of little value in evaluating PTH. Abnormalities are often present immediately after injury, but rapidly normalize within minutes to weeks and do not predict outcome.

Brainstem auditory evoked potentials are abnormal among groups of patients with head injury and post-concussion syndrome. These group differences are not useful in evaluating individual patients or predicting outcomes. Short-latency somatosensory evoked potentials are not valuable in evaluating patients with head injury.

Neuropsychological testing

Neuropsychological testing in head injury patients is often markedly abnormal in the acute phase, but often improves or resolves with the passage of time. The abnormalities are found in information processing, auditory vigilance, reaction time, sustained divided and distributed attention, visual and verbal memory, design fluency imagination, and analytic capacity. Studies suggest that functional recovery occurs sequentially following head injury, with attention and concentration improving first (within 6 months) and information processing last (after 12 months).

Relationship between cranial trauma and headache

Migraine, cluster headache, or chronic daily headache can occur after even trivial head injury. However, PTH is more common among patients with a history of headache. It usually lasts for 3–5 years, then abates independent of financial compensation. The IHS set a limit that the headache should come on within 2 weeks of head injury, which, while it is an arbitrary criterion, is useful in practice. If cranial trauma induces a headache process, it seems likely that it would have a relatively short latency. Certainly, it is difficult to accept the concept that a headache that starts years after cranial trauma is related to the trauma.

Diagnosis

The diagnosis of PTH and post-traumatic syndrome is established by an onset that is related to trauma and symptoms that are consistent with the syndrome. The differential diagnosis includes:

- subdural or epidural haematoma;
- CSF hypotension;
- cerebral vein thrombosis;
- cavernous sinus thrombosis;
- cervical or carotid artery dissection;
- cerebral haemorrhage;
- epilepsy; and
- hydrocephalus.

Management

The clinical syndrome dictates the management of PTH. Careful history, physical examination, and neuroimaging rule out structural problems such as low CSF pressure due to dural tears or chronic subdural haematoma. Since these patients are often misunderstood and distressed, they require support, an objective and comprehensive approach to treatment, and reassurance that the syndrome is a recognized one.

Primary headache syndromes, such as migraine, cluster, or chronic daily headache, that are triggered by cranial trauma are managed in the usual way. Cervical and soft-tissue injuries, anxiety, depression, and cognitive dysfunction should be identified and treated. We find valproate (divalproex) and tricyclic antidepressants, such as amitriptyline and imipramine, useful in treating PTH. Medication overuse can complicate treatment. The most effective tool is a straightforward explanation that pain-producing structures in the brain 'wind themselves up' to produce pain that was initially triggered by the trauma, but persists independent of the injury.

The triptans (sumatriptan, zolmitriptan, rizatriptan, and naratriptan) are effective for the migrainous exacerbation of PTH, but not for the baseline headache. Intravenous dihydroergotamine, repeated as needed, is effective for PTH that meets the criteria of chronic daily headache. Intravenous chlorpromazine has been effective in acute PTH. Analgesics and/or ergotamine overuse by patients with daily or near-daily headache should be identified if present and avoided if not. In general, abortive (acute) medications should be limited and preventive medications used preferentially. Physical therapy, exercise, chiropractic treatment, and massage have benefited some patients, particularly when the headache is related to cervical trauma. Other treatments that have not been rigorously tested but might improve function (especially in the acute phase) include heat, cold, electrotherapy, and cervical orthoses.

In the post-traumatic patient, two processes may occur simultaneously. The first, diffuse axonal injury, may occur because of acceleration and/or deceleration of the brain relative to the skull. When this is severe, it may be associated with abnormal MRI, positron emission spectroscopy, single photon emission computed tomography, and certain neuropsychological tests. The patient often improves over several months, and the tests often normalize. A second process, separate from the diffuse axonal injury, may be responsible for persistent headache, psychopathology, and neurocognitive deficits. This process may depend upon some not-yet-determined pre-existing factor or vulnerability required for the process to present itself fully in the individual.

The prognosis for PTH is uncertain because of difficulties with study designs. However, approximately one-third of patients are unable to return to work after head injury.

Summary

- Mild-to-moderate closed head trauma can trigger typical primary headaches, such as migraine, tension-type, cluster, and various forms of chronic daily headache.
- Women, older people, and patients whose heads were inclined or rotated at impact or who have had a rear-end collision in a vehicle are at the greatest risk for a poor outcome.
- Drug treatment, physical modalities, and supportive explanations are beneficial to patients with post-traumatic head injuries.

Further reading

Elson LM, Ward CC. Mechanisms and pathophysiology of mild head injury. *Semin Neurol* 1994; 14: 8–18.

Evans RW. The postconcussion syndrome and the sequelae of mild head injury. *Neurol Clin* 1992; 10: 815–47.

Gennarelli TA. Mechanisms of brain injury. *J Emerg Med* 1993; 1: 5–11.

Headache Classification Committee of the International Headache Society. Classification and diagnostic criteria for headache disorders, cranial neuralgias and facial pain. *Cephalalgia* 1988; 88(7): S1–96.

Jennett B, Frankowski RF. The epidemiology of head injury. In: Braakman R (ed). *Handbook of Clinical Neurology*. New York: Elsevier, 1990; 57: 1–16.

Lance JW, Goadsby PJ. *Mechanism and Management of Headache*, 6th edn. London: Butterworth–Heinemann, 1998.

Russell MB, Olesen J. Migraine associated with head trauma and its relation to migraine. *Eur J Neurol* 1996; 3: 424–8.

Schoenhuber R, Gentilini M. Neurophysiologic assessment of mild head injury. In: Levin HS, Eisenberg HM, Benton AL (eds). *Mild Head Injury*. New York: Oxford University Press, 1989: 142–50.

Ward C. Status of head injury modeling. Head and neck injury criteria. Washington DC: US Department of Transportation, 1981.

Young WB, Packard PC. Post-traumatic headache. In: Silberstein SD, Goadsby P (eds). *Headache*. Newton: Butterworth–Heinemann, 1997: 253–278.

11 Headache associated with disease in the intracranial cavity

Introduction

Headache is a common clinical manifestation of diseases that occur in the intracranial cavity. These disorders often alter intracranial pressure, either by acting as a mass or by disrupting the production, flow, or absorption of the cerebrospinal fluid (CSF). Clinical syndromes include post-lumbar puncture headache, spontaneous intracranial hypotension, idiopathic intracranial hypertension (IIH), brain tumour, hydrocephalus, intracranial haemorrhage, and subdural haematoma. The International Headache Society (IHS) calls this group of disorders 'headache associated with non-vascular intracranial disorders'. Diagnostic criteria are summarized in Table 11.1. Intracranial disease may lead to a worsening of a pre-existing headache type or to a new form of headache.

Cerebrospinal fluid

Cerebrospinal fluid production, flow, absorption, and pressure

CSF is produced primarily by the choroid plexus of the lateral ventricle. Humans produce about 500 ml/day of CSF, all of which is replaced every 6–8 hours. The factors that determine CSF pressure are listed in Table 11.2. Of these, transmitted venous pressure is the most important. Intracranial pressure can be elevated by any of the mechanisms listed in Table 11.3. For example, a mass lesion can produce elevated intracranial pressure when it reaches a critical size, obstructs the intracranial venous system to produce increased venous pressure, or obstructs the CSF pathways. Any increase in intracranial volume leads to increased intracranial pressure. Since an adult's skull is rigid, it forms a closed chamber, from which the foramen magnum is the only way by which CSF can exit into the vertebral canal.

When a patient who has low CSF pressure (intracranial hypotension) stands up, the intracranial pressure decreases more than it would if the pressure were normal to begin with. This pro-

Table 11.1 *Headache associated with non-vascular intracranial disorder: diagnostic criteria*

- Symptoms and/or signs of intracranial disorder
- Confirmation by appropriate investigation
- Headache as a new symptom or of a new type occurs temporally related to an intracranial disorder

Table 11.2 *Factors that determine CSF pressure*

- CSF secretion pressure
- CSF absorption rate
- Intracranial arterial pressure
- Intracranial venous pressure
- Brain bulk
- Hydrostatic pressure
- Presence of intact/surrounding coverings

Table 11.3 *Mechanisms for elevated intracranial pressure*

- Increased CSF production or secretion pressure
- Decreased CSF absorption
- Increased venous pressure
- Obstruction of normal CSF flow
- Increase in brain bulk: mass lesion/cerebral oedema
- Increased bulk or pressure in dura
- Combination of above

duces downward displacement of the brain and increased traction on the supporting structures of the brain (the dura mater, blood vessels, and dural sinuses). The consequence is a headache that may occur only when the patient is in the upright position. Secondary compensatory venous dilation may also contribute to the headache.

Intracranial hypotension (low CSF pressure)

Of the clinical symptoms of intracranial hypotension (Table 11.4), headache is the most common and almost inevitable feature. The headaches

● **Table 11.4** Features of low CSF pressure headache

- Pain: aggravated by upright position; relieved with recumbency. Aggravated by head shaking and jugular compression.
- Associated symptoms: nausea, vomiting, dizziness, tinnitus, photophobia, anorexia, and generalized malaise.
- Physical examination: within normal limits (rare neck stiffness, slow pulse rate 'vagus pulse').
- Lumbar puncture: opening pressure from 0 to 2.9 kPa (0 to 30 mmH$_2$O) CSF in the lateral decubitus position.

● **Table 11.5** Causes of low pressure headache syndrome

- **Spontaneous intracranial hypotension**
- **Symptomatic**

    Lumbar puncture: diagnostic, myelographic, and spinal anaesthesia

    Traumatic: head or back trauma
    　With CSF leak (dural tear, traumatic nerve root avulsion)
    　Without CSF leak

    Postoperative: craniotomy, spinal surgery, post-pneumonectomy (thoracoarachnoid fistula)
    　With CSF leak
    　Without CSF leak

    Spontaneous CSF leak: CSF rhinorrhoea, occult pituitary tumour, dural tear

    Systemic illnesses: dehydration, diabetic coma, hyperpnoea, meningoencephalitis, uraemia, severe systemic infection

may be frontal, occipital, or diffuse, and severe, dull, or throbbing. The headache is worse when the patient is in the erect position and relieved when the patient lies down. The pain is aggravated by head-shaking, Valsalva manoeuvre (coughing, straining, or sneezing), and jugular compression, and is not usually relieved with analgesics. The physical examination is usually normal; however, mild neck stiffness and a slow pulse rate (vagus pulse) may be present. The spinal fluid pressure usually ranges from 0 to 6.8 kPa (0 to 70 mmH$_2$O) and may be difficult to measure. The CSF composition is usually normal, but there may be slight protein elevation and a few blood cells in the fluid.

Intracranial hypotension can be divided into two categories (Table 11.5):

- spontaneous – no evidence of a CSF leak or systemic illness; and
- symptomatic – may be associated with a CSF leak.

The IHS classifies low CSF pressure headache as one that occurs or worsens less than 15 minutes after sitting up and disappears or improves less than 30 minutes after lying down. In clinical practice, headache with postural features should be considered because the diagnosis is missed if this possibility is not actively pursued.

Lumbar puncture is the most common cause of symptomatic intracranial hypotension, presumably because a CSF leak has occurred. Other causes include tears of the dura or nerve root sheath as a result of head or back trauma, craniotomy, or spinal surgery. Craniotomy or trauma can produce intracranial hypotension without a CSF leak by decreasing cerebral blood flow or the rate of CSF formation. Also, CSF rhinorrhoea (leading to a low pressure syndrome) may arise as a sequela of head injury or surgery, may be from a pituitary tumour, or no cause may be identifiable. Dehydration, hyperpnoea, meningoencephalitis, uraemia, severe systemic infection, and infusion of hypertonic solution can all cause CSF hypotension. Postural headache can also occur in patients who have had CSF shunts if the valve pressure is too low.

The syndrome of spontaneous intracranial hypotension resembles that of post-lumbar puncture headache in its clinical features. By definition, there are no identifiable causes of low CSF pressure. Three possible mechanisms have been proposed – decreased CSF production, increased CSF absorption, and CSF leakage from unidentified dural tears.

Many experts believe that occult CSF leakage is the major cause of low CSF pressure, and often the patient has a history of minor trauma (for example, falling, twisting, or stretching), vigorous exercise, strenuous effort, or sudden bouts of sneezing or coughing. Since the neurological examination is normal and headache is such a common complaint, the true incidence of spontaneous low CSF pressure is unknown.

Headache is the most common complication of lumbar puncture; it occurs in 15–30% of patients, and usually starts within the first few days after the procedure. This headache is especially common in younger patients, women, and those with a prior history of headache. Headache incidence varies according to the reason for the lumbar puncture. The syndrome occurs with surgical lumbar puncture (13%), obstetrical lumbar puncture (18%), and diagnostic lumbar puncture (32%; Table 11.6). No evidence supports the theory that keeping the patient supine after a lumbar puncture prevents a headache; in fact, prolonged recumbency may increase the risk of headache. A needle smaller than 22 gauge may decrease the incidence of headache, but a needle this small is difficult to use. Recently, a non-traumatic needle was recommended, and has resulted in a lower incidence of post-lumbar puncture headache. We recommend keeping patients relatively inactive by having them lie down for no more than 2–4 hours after the lumbar puncture, followed by mobilization. Using a non-traumatic needle may be advisable for a high-risk patient.

The patient who has an orthostatic headache that is exacerbated by becoming upright and relieved by lying down must be distinguished from the patient who has a headache that is aggravated by movement. If the headache is orthostatic, but the patient does not have orthostatic hypotension, the diagnosis is most likely intracranial hypotension (causes listed in Table 11.5). The diagnosis of low CSF pressure headache is made by the presence of an orthostatic headache for which there is an obvious cause, such as head or back trauma, a recent lumbar puncture, or a recent craniotomy. If no cause is apparent, lumbar puncture following normal computed tomography (CT) or magnetic resonance imaging (MRI) is indicated to document low CSF pressure. If the cause of the low pressure is known, the physician should proceed with the appropriate treatment. If the cause is uncertain, cisternography or ionic myelography to identify CSF leaks and a search for occult CSF rhinorrhoea can establish cause. This often requires referral to a neurologist or neurological surgeon.

Neuroimaging

Both CT and MRI are useful to evaluate patients with low-pressure headaches. They detect subdural haematomas caused by tears in bridging veins associated with intracranial hypotension. Also, MRI with gadolinium contrast often shows

● **Table 11.6** *Post-lumbar puncture headache*

Contributing factors

Prior headache
Female sex
Type of procedure

Non-contributing factors

Race
Quantity of CSF removed
Bloody tap
Multiple perforations of the dura?
Qualifications of the operator?

● **Table 11.7** *Treatment of low CSF headache*

- Bedrest
- Abdominal binder
- Caffeine
- Corticosteroids
- Epidural blood patch
- Continuous epidural saline infusion

diffuse meningeal enhancement (DME), which occurs with all types of low CSF pressure headache and can be confused with an inflammatory process. These studies should be carried out prior to a lumbar puncture because DME may be seen after an uncomplicated lumbar puncture.

Treatment

Treatment for intracranial hypotension may include bedrest, peripheral intravascular volume expansion, corticosteroids, caffeine, a blood patch, an abdominal binder, and continuous intrathecal saline infusion (Table 11.7). The treatment should be based on the aetiology (*see* Table 11.5). Associated illnesses should be treated, and if a CSF leak exists, it should be repaired if it can be identified and is accessible. Treatments of post-lumbar puncture headache and spontaneous intracranial hypotension are similar. Post-craniotomy hypotension is not discussed here.

Treatment begins with the non-invasive modalities of bedrest and an abdominal binder (Table 11.7). If the patient does not improve, intravenous (i.v.) or oral caffeine can be used. This causes intracerebral arterial constriction and may produce significant relief. In one study (Silberstein, Marcelis),

500 mg of i.v. caffeine sodium benzoate was dramatically effective in 75% of patients with low CSF pressure who had undergone previous lumbar puncture. A second dose 2 hours later raised the success rate to 85%. In an open study, 2 l of intravenous Ringer's lactate solution that contained 500 mg of caffeine sodium benzoate was given at a rate of 1 l for the first hour and then 1 l over 2 hours. This could be repeated after 4 hours if the patient continued to have symptoms. The total response rate in 18 patients was 75%.

In a placebo-controlled, double-blind study, 40 postpartum patients who had post-lumbar puncture headache were given oral caffeine (300 mg) – 120% of the dose of caffeine in caffeine sodium benzoate (250 mg caffeine, 250 mg sodium benzoate). Beneficial effects were rapid, with 70% of patients experiencing relief within 4 hours and no symptom recurrence.

A brief trial of corticosteroids may be beneficial. If relief is not obtained within 24 hours, a quick corticosteroid taper is recommended because of potential side effects. If the patient continues to be symptomatic after a non-invasive medical approach, a blood patch is indicated. With a 90% success rate, the blood patch is the most successful treatment for low CSF pressure headache. Studies indicate that no major complications result, and the symptoms of injection site pain, leg pain, and weakness are mild and transient. An anaesthesiologist typically performs a blood patch by infusing 10–20 ml of the patient's own blood in the lumbar epidural space under sterile conditions. The presumed mechanism of action of the blood patch is an immediate gelatinous tamponade of a dural leak, followed by fibrin deposition and fibroblastic activity.

Increased intracranial pressure

Many disorders are associated with the syndrome of increased intracranial pressure (Table 11.8). Correlating clinical features with underlying pathology is difficult because increased intracranial pressure is not always associated with headache or papilloedema, and no direct correlation exists between the degree of pressure elevation and the presence of headache.

Table 11.8 Syndromes of increased intracranial pressure

Primary

Idiopathic intracranial hypertension with papilloedema

Idiopathic intracranial hypertension without papilloedema

Secondary

Hydrocephalus

Mass lesion
neoplasm
stroke – haematoma

Meningitis/encephalitis

Trauma

Major intracranial and extracranial venous obstruction

Drugs: vitamin A, nalidixic acid, anabolic steroids, steroid withdrawal

Systemic disease: renal disease, hypoparathyroidism, systemic lupus erythematosus

Table 11.9 Mechanisms for headache with increased intracranial pressure

- Traction on pain-sensitive intracerebral vessels (venous sinuses and arteries at the base of the brain)
- Transient herniation of hippocampal gyri
- Traction on cranial or cervical nerves, or elevation of intracranial pressure

Headaches do not usually occur with mild-to-moderate pressure elevations unless there is traction or distortion of pain-sensitive structures; the notable exceptions occur with acute hydrocephalus and IIH.

The postulated mechanisms for increased intracranial pressure headache are listed in Table 11.9. In the setting of mass lesions, several pain mechanisms may operate. For example, a convexity meningioma may distort the adjacent middle meningeal artery and cause pain, which may be referred to the ipsilateral frontotemporal region (Figure 11.1). The meningioma may also act as a mass lesion, increasing intracranial pressure or producing traction on intracranial nerves. The rate of change in pressure may be critical. Sudden increases caused by tumours that obstruct the foramen of Monro or the cerebral aqueduct may result in abrupt, severe headache and gait disturbance, syncope, incontinence, or visual disturbance.

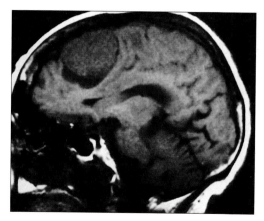

● *Figure 11.1* *Meningioma.*

Intracranial neoplasms

Headache occurs at presentation in about half of patients with brain tumours, and it develops in the course of the disease in 60% of patients. In contrast, brain tumour as a cause of headache is rare. One pre-CT pre-MRI survey of 778 patients with cerebral tumour indicated that headache was the earliest or principal symptom in 54% of patients. Later studies using neuroimaging show that headache is less likely to be an initial symptom of brain tumour, because of the earlier detection by and relatively easy access to neuroimaging. Elevation of intracranial pressure is not necessary to produce headache. The headache is usually bilateral, but it may be more prominent or confined to the side of the tumour. The headache's location is sometimes, but not always, dependent on the tumour's location. Supratentorial tumours may produce frontotemporal radiation (ophthalmic division of the trigeminal nerve). Infratentorial tumours may produce occipital nuchal pain (IX and X cranial nerves).

In a series of 111 patients whose diagnosis of primary (34%) or metastatic (66%) brain tumour was made by neuroimaging, 48% had headache. The headache was similar to tension-type headache in 77% of the patients, to migraine in 9%, and to other headache types in 14%. Unlike true tension-type headaches, brain tumour headaches worsened by bending in 32% of patients, and nausea or vomiting was present in 40%. Patients with a history of prior headache were more likely to have brain tumour headache and, in many cases, its character was similar to, but more severe than, that of the patient's prior headache.

Headache is more common as a symptom of brain tumour in children (over 90%) than in adults (around 60%). Perhaps this is explained in part by the greater frequency of posterior fossa tumours in children – tumours in this location are more likely to cause headache. Most children with headache from brain tumour (94%) have neurological signs, and in 96%, diagnostic clues appear within 4 months of the headache onset. Headache is rarely observed in the very young, perhaps because of the expansile nature of the infant skull or their inability to communicate.

Brain tumour headache can mimic migraine or tension-type headache. Therefore, a headache of recent onset, or one that has changed in character or is accompanied by a neurological sign or symptom that is not a migraine aura, requires a thorough evaluation, especially if the headache is severe or occurs with nausea or vomiting. In other space-occupying lesions, such as subdural haematomas and brain abscesses, headache is an earlier and more frequent symptom than for brain tumours. This is believed to be because of the more rapid evolution and greater extent of these lesions.

Intracranial hypertension

Intracranial hypertension may be either *idiopathic*, with no clear identifiable cause, or *symptomatic*, a result of venous sinus occlusion, radical neck dissection, hypoparathyroidism, vitamin A intoxication, systemic lupus, renal disease, or drug side effects (nalidixic acid, danocrine, steroid withdrawal; Table 11.8). It occurs at a rate of one case per 100,000 per year in the general population, and 19.3 cases per 100,000 per year in obese women of age 20–50 years.

The syndrome of IIH (also called 'pseudotumour cerebri' or 'benign intracranial hypertension') is a condition of increased intracranial pressure of unknown cause that occurs predominantly in obese women of childbearing age (Table 11.10). Before a definitive diagnosis can be made, the physician must exclude brain tumours and other intracranial mass lesions, infections, hypertensive encephalopathy, pulmonary encephalopathy (related to chronic carbon dioxide toxicity), and obstruction of the cerebral ventricles. The symptoms of IIH are those of generalized increased intracranial pressure, with

127

> ● **Table 11.10** *Features of idiopathic intracranial hypertension*
>
> - Headache: chronic tension-type headache with migrainous features, may be present upon awakening. Can be intermittent or absent.
> - Associated features: pulsatile tinnitus, transient visual obscurations, diplopia, visual loss, shoulder and arm pain.
> - Patients: predominantly obese women aged 20–50 years.
> - Physical and neurological examination: within normal limits, excpt for papilloedema, visual loss, obesity, VIth nerve palsy.
> - Neuroradiology: CT or MRI show no evidence of intracranial mass, hydrocephalus, or venous sinus thrombosis. (Empty sella may be present.)
> - Lumbar puncture: demonstrates increased CSF pressure with a normal composition. (May show decreased protein.)
> - No other causes of increased CSF pressure present.

headache occurring in most, but not all, patients. Unilateral, bilateral, frontal, or occipital headache may occur, although bifrontotemporal headache is the most common. Transient visual clouding in one or both eyes, which usually lasts for seconds, occurs with all forms of increased intracranial pressure with papilloedema. Other common symptoms include pulsatile tinnitus, diplopia, and visual loss. Some patients report retro-orbital pain as well as shoulder and arm pain. Signs include papilloedema and VIth nerve palsy. The patient is commonly a young, obese woman with chronic daily headaches who has normal laboratory studies, a normal neurological examination (except for papilloedema), and an empty sella (Table 11.10, Figures 11.2 and 11.3).

Symptomatic intracranial hypertension can be secondary to changes in cranial venous outflow, which may influence intracranial pressure by increasing cerebral blood volume, producing brain oedema, and impairing CSF absorption. Intracranial venous outflow obstruction can be caused by chronic otitis, head trauma, tumours, hypercoaguable states, and cerebral oedema. Extracranial venous outflow obstruction occurs with surgical ligation and further compression of venous outflow. Cranial venous outflow hypertension can also occur without obstruction in patients with arteriovenous malformations (AVMs), cardiac failure, and pulmonary failure.

The cause of IIH is unknown. Postulated mechanisms are listed in Table 11.11. Patients are not particularly ill, although their headaches may be very severe. Somnolence, fever, or other systemic symptoms suggest venous sinus occlusion or some other cause of increased pressure. If the patient has a history of headache, the headaches of IIH may be similar in quality, but more constant and severe. The headaches are usually daily and continuous, qualifying as chronic daily headache. Pain on eye movement, not a common feature of migraine, occurs in up to 20% of patients with IIH. Another feature, cranial bruit, may be audible to observers, and is caused by turbulence in the major venous sinuses. This pulse-synchronous, pulsatile noise stops with carotid compression.

Papilloedema is occasionally found while patients are being examined for another purpose, and 5–10% of patients are asymptomatic. Loss of visual field and visual acuity is the only significant complication of IIH with papilloedema.

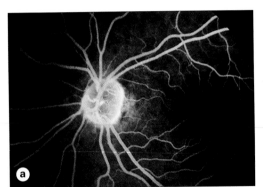 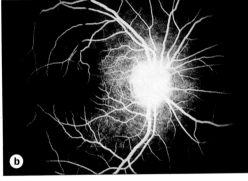

● **Figure 11.2** *Fluoroscein anglography of fundi (a) Normal (b) Papilloedema.*

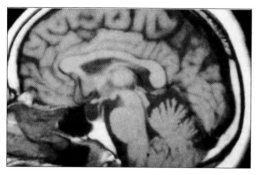

● *Figure 11.3* *Empty sella.*

● *Table 11.11* *Pathophysiology of idiopathic intracranial hypertension*

- Increased rate of CSF formation
- Increased intracranial venous pressure
- Decreased rate of CSF absorption
- Increase in brain interstitial fluid (oedema)

Ophthalmological examination should include intraocular pressure, visual fields, optic disc photos, visual acuity, and a search for a relative afferent pupil (one that reacts more to light shined into the other eye than to light shined directly into itself).

Idiopathic intracranial hypertension without papilloedema

Intracranial hypertension can occur without papilloedema. The clinical, historical, radiographic, and demographic characteristics are identical to those of patients with papilloedema except for:

- possible association with prior head trauma or meningitis;
- extended delay in diagnosis (which requires lumbar puncture in the absence of papilloedema); and
- no evidence of visual loss as seen in patients with IIH with papilloedema.

Patients, particularly obese women, with chronic daily headache and symptoms of increased intracranial pressure (i.e. pulsatile tinnitus, a history of head trauma or meningitis, an empty sella on neuroimaging studies, or a headache that is unrelieved by standard therapy) should have a diagnostic lumbar puncture.

Treatment

Treatment of elevated intracranial pressure depends on the underlying cause. In many cases, the history, clinical examination, and neuroradiographical studies may define the syndrome, with distinctive therapy preceding further diagnostic studies. Thus, arteriovenous malformation, abscess, cerebral neoplasm, cerebral infarct, acute meningitis, subarachnoid haemorrhage (SAH), subdural haematoma, and acute obstructive hydrocephalus may be treated surgically (drainage, shunt) or medically (antibiotics, hyperventilation, corticosteroids, hypertonic osmotic diuretics).

For patients with IIH (with or without papilloedema) and chronic meningitis, and for some cases of SAH, diagnosis is based on neuroimaging (with attention to empty sella and sinus thrombosis), followed by a lumbar puncture. If the lumbar puncture is unremarkable and intracranial pressure is greater than 19.6 kPa (200 mmH$_2$O) in non-obese patients, then IIH is the likely diagnosis

Once the diagnosis of IIH is made, secondary causes should be sought and eliminated. More than 50 diseases, conditions, toxins, or pharmaceuticals (including megadoses of vitamin A) have been claimed to be associated with this condition (*see* Table 11.8). However, in a sex- and age-matched case control study, no evidence was found to associate IIH with pregnancy, hypertension, diabetes, thyroid disease, iron deficiency anaemia, or the use of tetracyclines or oral contraceptives. Obesity and weight gain were more common in the IIH group – obese patients should be encouraged to lose weight. If the patient is asymptomatic and has no visual loss, no treatment is indicated, but careful ophthalmological follow-up is needed. If there is no papilloedema or visual loss and the only complaint is headache, then the patient should be treated aggressively.

Headache associated with IIH with papil-loedema frequently responds to standard treatment (Table 11.12). These patients require careful neurological and ophthalmological follow-up (including visual fields) because the major comorbidity of this disorder is blindness. Treatment options include repeated lumbar punctures, carbonic anhydrase inhibitors, and other diuretics. Intractable cases may require a lumboperitoneal or ventriculoperitoneal shunt. Visual loss as a result of papilloedema can be treated with optic nerve sheath fenestration.

> **Table 11.12** Treatment of idiopathic intracranial hypertension
>
> - Eliminate symptomatic causes
> - Weight loss if obese
> - Standard headache treatment
> - Carbonic anhydrase inhibitors and loop diuretics
> - Short course of high-dose corticosteroids
> - Serial lumbar punctures
> - Lumboperitoneal or ventriculoperitoneal shunt
> - Optic nerve sheath fenestration

Exertional and cough headaches

While coughing and exertion rarely provoke headache, these activities can aggravate any type of headache. However, transient, severe head pain upon coughing, sneezing, weight-lifting, bending, straining at stool, or stooping defines cough headache. Cough headache, which is uncommon, mainly affects middle-aged men and runs its course over a few years. The most recent IHS classification (Tables 11.13 and 11.14) separates benign cough headache and benign exertional headache, since these have different clinical features, diagnostic evaluation, and treatment responses.

Headache associated with sexual activity may be precipitated by masturbation or coitus. Benign sexual headache is now a well-defined entity, with three types recognized (Table 11.15). The most frequent is the explosive type, which begins suddenly at the time of orgasm and is thought to be related to haemodynamic changes. Patients often have coexistent exertional headaches.

> **Table 11.13** Benign cough headache
>
> - Benign cough headache is a bilateral headache of sudden onset, lasting less than 1 minute, precipitated by coughing.
> - It may be prevented by avoiding coughing.
> - It may be diagnosed only after structural lesions such as posterior fossa tumour have been excluded by neuroimaging.

> **Table 11.14** Benign exertional headache
>
> - Benign exertional headache is specifically brought on by physical exercise.
> - It is bilateral, throbbing in nature at onset, and may develop migrainous features in patients susceptible to migraine.
> - It lasts from 5 minutes to 24 hours.
> - It is prevented by avoiding excessive exertion, particularly in hot weather or at high altitude.
> - It is not associated with any systemic or intracranial disorder.

Benign cough headache

The mean age of onset of this infrequent headache type is 55 years (range 19–73 years), but it is twice as common in patients over 40 years of age. Benign cough headache is four times more common in men than in women. The pain is severe, usually bilateral, with a bursting or explosive quality that lasts a few seconds or minutes. Bending or lying down may be impossible. The neurological examination is usually normal. Because the headache is not usually associated with nausea or vomiting, vomiting suggests an organic basis. About 25% of patients have an antecedent respiratory infection. Most patients are pain-free between attacks, but dull, aching pain may persist for hours following the paroxysms. As these patients often complain of a continuous headache, the physician should ask if exertion is a trigger. The long-term outlook for such patients is favourable. Many respond dramatically to indomethacin, 25–50 mg three times a day. Some patients have prolonged relief following a lumbar puncture.

Symptomatic cough headache

Patients with symptomatic cough headache are significantly younger than are those with benign cough headache (Table 11.16). In addition to coughing, this headache can be precipitated by

● **Table 11.15** *Headache associated with sexual activity*

Headache is:

- precipitated by sexual excitement,
- bilateral at onset,
- prevented or eased by ceasing sexual activity before orgasm,
- not associated with any intracranial disorder such as aneurysm.

Dull type
  A dull ache in the head and neck that intensifies as sexual excitement increases.

Explosive type
  A sudden severe ('explosive') headache occurring at orgasm.

Postural type
  Postural headache resembling that of low CSF pressure developing after coitus.

laughing, weight-lifting, or acute body or head postural changes. Symptomatic cough headache, unlike the benign variety, can be caused by a hindbrain abnormality, posterior fossa meningioma, midbrain cyst, basilar impression, acoustic neurinoma, brain tumour, or an Arnold–Chiari malformation. Symptomatic cough headache does not respond to indomethacin. If a patient does not respond to indomethacin, has posterior fossa signs (such as ataxia or double vision), or is younger than 50 years of age, MRI must be carried out.

Cough headache can be confused with other disorders, such as exertional headache, effort migraine, and coital headache.

Benign exertional headache

Benign exertional headache onset ranges from 10–48 years of age, which is about 40 years earlier than benign cough headache onset. The headache is typically throbbing, lasts from 5 minutes to 24 hours, and is provoked by physical exercise. The pain usually begins during exertion, is non-explosive, and can be either bilateral or unilateral. Unlike benign cough headache, it often responds to standard migraine treatments.

Symptomatic exertional headache

Symptomatic exertional headache usually is explosive, severe, and bilateral at onset. Causes may include SAH, sinusitis, and brain mass.

Benign sexual headache

Benign sexual headache is a disorder of middle life (24–57 years of age). The pain is usually bilateral, severe, and explosive, with occasional throbbing and stabbing. Its duration ranges from less than 1 minute to 3 hours (average 30 minutes). The frequency of episodes relates directly to sexual intercourse or masturbation; up to one-third of patients have similar episodes with physical exertion.

● **Table 11.16** *Cough, exertional, and sexual headache*

Parameter	Cough headache		Exertional headache		Sexual headache	
	Benign	**Symptomatic**	**Benign**	**Symptomatic**	**Benign**	**Symptomatic**
Patients (n)	13	17	16	12	13	1
Age, range (years)	67 ± 11, 44–81	39 ± 14, 15–63	24 ± 11, 10–48	42 ± 14, 18–61	41 ± 9, 24–57	60
Sex (% men)	77	59	88	43	85	100
Duration	Seconds to 30 minutes	Seconds to days	Minutes to 2 days	1 day to 1 month	1 minute to 3 hours	10 days
Bilateral localization (%)	92	94	56	100	77	Yes
Quality	Sharp, stabbing	Bursting, stabbing	Pulsating	Explosive, pulsating	Explosive + pulsating	Explosive + pulsating
Other manifestations	No	Posterior fossa signs	Nausea, photophobia	Nausea, vomiting, double vision, neck rigidity	None	Vomiting, neck rigidity
Diagnosis	Idiopathic	Chiari Type I malformation	Idiopathic	SAH, sinusitis, brain metastases	Idiopathic	SAH

Modified from Pascual et al., 1996.

Symptomatic sexual headache

Explosive headache that occurs during coitus can also be a symptom of SAH. One pre-CT era study of 103 patients emphasized the importance of careful evaluation for organic disease in patients with exertional headache. The largest series of benign and symptomatic headaches of sudden onset provoked by cough, physical exercise, or sexual excitement concluded that:

- symptomatic cough headache began earlier, lasted longer, and was more frequent than benign cough headache;
- most common cause of symptomatic cough headache was Chiari type I malformation;
- causes of symptomatic exertional headache were SAH, sinusitis, and brain masses;
- symptomatic exertional and sexual headaches began later in life and lasted longer than the benign variety;
- all patients with symptomatic exertional and sexual headaches had manifestations of meningeal irritation or intracranial hypertension; and
- patients with subarachnoid bleeding had only one headache episode.

Neuroradiological studies do not need to be carried out for patients who have:

- clinically typical benign sexual or exertional headaches (men around 30–40 years of age);
- normal examination;
- short-duration, multiple episodes of pulsating pain; and
- pain that responds to ergotamine, triptans, or preventive migraine treatment.

All other patients must have a brain CT (and a CSF examination if the CT scan is normal).

Benign cough and exertional headaches were formerly thought to be similar conditions. However, they have different triggers, age of onset, and duration and quality of attack, and they respond differently to treatment.

Summary

- Headache is a common manifestation of high or low intracranial pressure caused by disruption of CSF production, flow, or absorption.
- Migraine or tension-type headaches are distinguished from headache caused by a brain tumour because of a change in the character of the patient's usual headaches or a neurological sign or symptom not easily explained by migraine aura. Patients with these changes require a thorough neurological evaluation.
- Benign exertional and sexual headache begin earlier in life than the symptomatic varieties. In contrast, symptomatic cough headaches begin earlier in life than the benign variety.

Further reading

Fishman RA. *Cerebrospinal Fluid in Diseases of the Nervous System*, 2nd edn. Philadelphia: WB Saunders, 1992.

Forsyth PA, Posner JB. Headaches in patients with brain tumors. A study of 111 patients. *Neurology* 1993; 43: 1678–83.

Gormley JB. Treatment of post-spinal headache. *Anesthesiology* 1960; 21: 565–6.

Lay CL, Campbell JK, Mokri B. Low cerebrospinal fluid pressure headache. In: Goadsby P, Silberstein SD (eds). *Blue Books of Practical Neurology: Headache*. Boston: Butterworth–Heinemann, 1997: 355–68.

Pascual J, Igelsias F, Oterino A, Vazques-Barquero A, Berciano J. Cough, exertional, and sexual headaches: an analysis of 72 benign and symptomatic cases. *Neurology* 1996; 46: 1520–4.

Silberstein SD. Drug induced headache. *Neurol Clin NA* 1998; 16(1): 107–23.

Silberstein SD, Marcelis J. Headache associated with abnormalities in intracranial structures or pressure including brain tumor and post-LP headache. In: Dalessio D, Silberstein SD (eds). *Wolff's Headache and Other Head Pain*, 6th edn. New York: Oxford University Press, 1993: 438–61.

Silberstein SD, Lipton RB, Goadsby PJ. *Headache in Clinical Practice*. Oxford: Isis Medical Media, 1997.

Wall M. The headache profile of idiopathic intracranial hypertension. *Cephalalgia* 1990; 10: 331–5.

12 Sinus headache

Sinusitis

Acute sinusitis, a relatively uncommon cause of headache in adults, results from infection of one or more of the cranial sinuses (Figure 12.1). Sinusitis is overdiagnosed as a cause of headache in adults based on the belief that pain over the sinuses must be related to the sinuses. In fact, frontal head pain is more often caused by migraine and tension-type headache. It follows that if a patient fails to respond to treatment, one should reconsider the diagnosis for sinus disease. Whether nasal obstruction can lead to chronic headache is controversial.

Acute sinusitis is usually characterized by purulent discharge in the nasal passages and a pain profile determined by the site of infection. Since sphenoid sinusitis differs from the other forms of sinusitis, both in clinical features and treatment, it is considered separately. Although it represents only 3% of sinusitis cases, sphenoid sinusitis is important out of proportion to its prevalence because it is potentially life-threatening.

In this chapter the relevant anatomy and pathophysiology of sinusitis, its clinical features, diagnostic testing, and treatment are discussed, and then sphenoidal sinusitis and nasal headache are described.

Anatomy and pathophysiology

Figure 12.2 illustrates the structure of the ostiomeatal complex of the nasal passages. The primary functions of the nasal passages are humidification, warming, and removal of particulate material from inspired air. The paranasal sinuses are air-filled cavities that communicate with the nasal airway. Any bacterial contamination of the sinuses is cleared by constant motion of the cilia and a mucous layer. Obstruction of the mucociliary flow or the sinus ostia causes oxygen partial pressure within the sinuses to decrease and carbon dioxide partial pressure to increase. This stagnant, anaerobic environment facilitates bacterial growth. Both aerobic and anaerobic bacteria play a role in chronic sinusitis. The ethmoid sinuses are key to sinus infection because their involvement can cause maxillary or frontal sinus involvement. Obstruction of the sinus ostia is the usual precursor to sinusitis. Although sinuses are relatively insensitive to pain, the pain associated with sinusitis comes from engorged and inflamed nasal structures – the nasofrontal ducts, turbinates, ostia, and superior nasal spaces.

The otolaryngological literature distinguishes between acute sinusitis (lasting from 1 day to 3 weeks), subacute sinusitis (lasting from 3 weeks to 3 months), and chronic sinusitis (lasting more

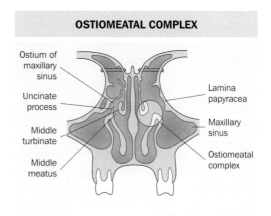

ANATOMY OF THE SINUSES

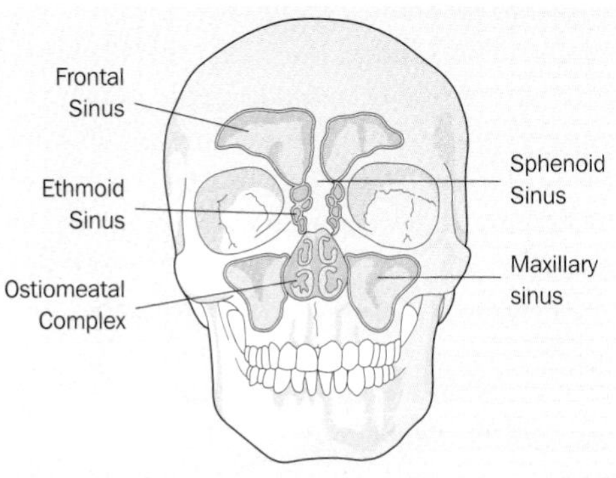

Frontal Sinus
Ethmoid Sinus
Ostiomeatal Complex
Sphenoid Sinus
Maxillary sinus

● *Figure 12.1* *The paranasal sinuses.*

OSTIOMEATAL COMPLEX

Ostium of maxillary sinus
Uncinate process
Middle turbinate
Middle meatus
Lamina papyracea
Maxillary sinus
Ostiomeatal complex

● *Figure 12.2* *Position of the region known as the ostiomeatal complex.*

than 3 months). Of these, only acute sinusitis is universally accepted as a cause of head and face pain (Table 12.1). With the exception of sphenoidal sinusitis, purulent nasal discharge, occurring spontaneously or with suction, is a diagnostic hallmark. As discussed below, pathology should be evident on radiography, computed tomography (CT), magnetic resonance imaging (MRI), or endoscopy.

The pattern of pain is dictated by the location of the sinus disease. Maxillary sinus pain is located mostly in the cheek, the gums, and the teeth of the upper jaw. Ethmoid sinusitis produces pain between the eyes with tenderness of the eyeball that is aggravated by eye movement. Frontal sinusitis produces pain mainly in the forehead, and sphenoid sinusitis produces pain at times in the vertex, but is generally localized. Ethmoid sinusitis and maxillary sinusitis are usually associated with rhinitis. Other symptoms and signs include facial pain, anosmia (inability to smell), pain with mastication, halitosis, fever, headache, and a history of respiratory infection. Headache associated with paranasal sinus disease usually has a deep, dull, aching quality combined with a heaviness and fullness. It is seldom associated with nausea and vomiting.

Sinus infections can result in several serious complications, including acute suppurative meningitis, a subdural or epidural abscess, or a brain abscess. In addition, osteomyelitis or subperiosteal abscess can occur. Infection of the ethmoid and sphenoid sinuses is responsible for orbital complications, which include oedema, orbital cellulitis, and subperiosteal and orbital abscesses. Migraine and tension-type headaches are often confused with true sinus headaches because the pain location is similar. The criteria for *acute* sinus headache, listed in Table 12.1, must be strictly fulfilled to diagnose International Headache Society (HIS) sinus headache. On the other hand, the relationship between headache and *subacute* and *chronic* sinus disease is unclear, and the IHS has not validated them as a cause of headache or facial pain unless the patient relapses into an acute stage.

Diagnostic testing

When sinusitis is suspected on clinical grounds, diagnostic testing is usually helpful. Air–fluid

● **Table 12.1** *Acute sinus headache.*
IHS diagnostic criteria

A Purulent discharge in the nasal passage, either spontaneous or by suction

B Pathological findings in one or more of the following tests:
- Radiographic examination
- Computed tomography or magnetic resonance imaging
- Transillumination

C Simultaneous onset of headache and sinusitis

D Headache location:
- In acute frontal sinusitis, headache is located directly over the sinus and may radiate to the vertex or behind the eyes
- In acute maxillary sinusitis, headache is located over the antral area and may radiate to the upper teeth or the forehead
- In acute ethmoiditis, headache is located between the eyes and may radiate to the temporal area
- In acute sphenoiditis, headache is located in the occipital area, the vertex, the frontal region, or behind the eyes

E Headache disappears after treatment of acute sinusitis

levels on standard skull and sinus films support the diagnosis. However, standard radiography does not adequately evaluate the anterior ethmoid air cells, the upper two-thirds of the nasal cavity, or the infundibular, middle meatus, and frontal recess air passages.

Computed tomography

Mucosal thickening, sclerosis, clouding, or air-fluid levels may be shown by CT. When imaging is performed in the coronal plane, it adequately demonstrates the ethmoid complex and can reveal the extent of mucosal disease in the ostiomeatal complex.

Magnetic resonance imaging

For detecting a fungal infection MRI is more sensitive than CT, although during the oedematous phase of the nasal cycle the image can falsely resemble pathological changes. Maxillary mucosal thickening of more than 6 mm, complete sinus opacification, and air–fluid levels on neuroimaging correlate with positive sinus cultures.

Transillumination, ultrasonography, and anterior rhinoscopy

Sinus transillumination and ultrasonography have poor sensitivity and specificity for the diagnosis. Routine anterior rhinoscopy performed with a headlight and nasal speculum allows only limited inspection of the anterior nasal cavity. These procedures have at best a minor role in the evaluation of patients for sinusitis.

Diagnostic fibreoptic endoscopy

Although not normally used by primary care physicians, flexible fibreoptic rhinoscopy is available in specialty clinics. It allows a direct view of the nasal passages and sinus drainage areas, and is complementary to CT or MRI. Easily performed and readily tolerated, the procedure facilitates culture and diagnosis if purulent material is seen in the sinus drainage region. Referral to an ear, nose, and throat specialist for endoscopy should be considered when a sinus-related problem is suspected, the patient has failed conservative medical treatment, and/or CT or MRI is inconclusive.

Treatment

Management goals for treating sinusitis include:

- treatment of bacterial infection;
- reduction of ostial swelling;
- sinus drainage; and
- maintenance of sinus ostia patency.

Uncomplicated sinusitis other than sphenoid sinusitis should be treated with a broad-spectrum oral antibiotic for 10–14 days. As nasal culture does not accurately predict sinus pathogens, the initial treatment is empirical. A 10-day course of amoxicillin is the first-line treatment of acute bacterial sinusitis. Co-trimoxazole (trimethoprim–sulfamethaxazole) can be considered as first-line therapy for patients who are allergic to penicillin. Beta-lactamase-resistant agents do not offer a significant advantage over amoxicillin. Many patients, even those who are proved to have a beta-lactamase-producing organism, respond to amoxicillin alone. Second-line therapy can be used if a patient is allergic or has not responded to first-line therapy. For second-line therapy, any agent with an approved indication for acute bacterial sinusitis, other than amoxicillin and co-trimoxazole, may be used.

Steam and saline prevent crusting of secretions and may facilitate mucociliary clearance. Locally active vasoconstrictor agents provide symptomatic relief by shrinking inflamed and swollen nasal mucosa. Their use should be limited to 3–4 days to prevent rebound vasodilation. Oral decongestants should be used if treatment for more than 3 days is necessary. These agents are α-adrenergic agonists that reduce nasal blood flow without the risk of rebound vasodilation. Antihistamines are not effective in the acute treatment of rhinitis. Anti-inflammatory topical corticosteroids may help maintain patency of the ostia.

Treatment failure and recurrent infections are indications for neuroimaging and endoscopy to search for a source of obstruction. A sinus culture should be considered. Endoscopic nasal surgery may be necessary to reopen and maintain the patency of the sinus ostia and ostiomeatal complex. Complications can be treated with high doses of intravenous antibiotics or surgical drainage of enclosed spaces.

Sphenoid sinusitis

Sphenoid sinusitis is discussed separately because of its unique clinical features, treatment, and complications. Although it is usually accompanied by pansinusitis, it can also occur alone. Sphenoid sinusitis is frequently misdiagnosed because the sphenoid sinus is not adequately seen on routine sinus radiographs and cannot be examined directly with a flexible endoscope. The sphenoid sinus is deep in the nasal cavity within the body of the sphenoid bone. As a result of its close proximity to the central venous system, cranial nerves, and meninges, infection may spread to these structures and present as a central nervous system infection or neurological catastrophe. This significant morbidity and mortality requires that the condition be identified early and managed aggressively.

Symptoms

Headache is an almost universal complaint among patients with acute sphenoid sinusitis. The headache is aggravated when the patient stands, walks, bends, or coughs. It often interferes with sleep and is poorly relieved by narcotics. Headache location varies. The 'classic' vertex headache is not as common as a frontal, occipital, or temporal headache, but most common is headache occurring in a combination of these regions. Periorbital pain is common. This contrasts with the common teaching that a retroorbital or vertex headache is the most common presenting symptom of sphenoid sinusitis. Nausea and vomiting frequently occur, but nasal discharge, stuffiness, and postnasal drip are unusual. Fever occurs in over half the patients.

Diagnosis

The diagnosis of sphenoid sinusitis is frequently delayed. It should be included in the differential diagnosis of acute or subacute headache. Sphenoid sinusitis may be mistaken for frontal or ethmoid sinusitis, aseptic meningitis, septic thrombophlebitis, or a brain abscess. It can mimic trigeminal neuralgia, migraine, a carotid artery aneurysm, or a brain tumour.

The clinical features of a severe, intractable, new-onset headache that interferes with sleep and is not relieved by simple analgesics should alert the physician to the possibility of sphenoid sinusitis. The headache increases in severity with the passage of time and has no specific location. Pain or paraesthesias in the facial distribution of the Vth nerve and photophobia or eye tearing are also suggestive of sphenoid sinusitis. The physical examination may not be helpful. Not all patients are febrile, sinus tenderness is rarely present, and pus is not always seen, although careful examination of the nose and throat often does reveal pus.

Neuroimaging is necessary to diagnose sphenoid sinusitis definitely. Some patients can be diagnosed using plain sinus radiography, but because of the superimposition of soft tissue, plain films are not diagnostic in 25% of cases. If sphenoid sinusitis is suspected and plain radiography is not diagnostic, CT or MRI is indicated (Figure 12.3).

Complications

Major complications of sphenoid sinusitis include bacterial meningitis, cavernous sinus thrombosis, subdural abscess, cortical vein thrombosis, ophthalmoplegia, and pituitary insufficiency. In addition, sphenoid sinusitis can present as aseptic meningitis because of the presence of a parameningeal focus (*see* Chapter 9).

Patients may present with the complications of sphenoid sinusitis – visual loss mimicking optic neuritis, multiple cranial nerve palsies, or papilloedema. Sudden onset that results from cavernous sinus thrombosis can mimic a subarachnoid haemorrhage.

Treatment

Sphenoid sinusitis without complications is managed with high-dose intravenous antibiotics and topical and systemic decongestants for 10–14 days. If the fever (if present) and the headache do not start to improve within 24–48 hours, or if any complications are present or develop, sphenoid sinus drainage is indicated.

Nasal headache

A septal deformity, especially one of traumatic origin, is believed by some investigators to exert pressure on the pain-sensitive structure of the lateral nasal wall, causing referred pain and 'chronic headache'. Several studies of this condition do not confirm the relationship between the headache onset and the development of nasal obstruction. Studies do suggest that about one-third of patients with nasal obstructions have headaches. Since the prevalence of migraine in the population is about 11%, episodic tension-type headache about 40%, and chronic tension-type headache 3%, these data are difficult to interpret. Of patients who had surgery to relieve nasal obstruction, headache relief was much more likely in those who also experienced relief of nasal congestion.

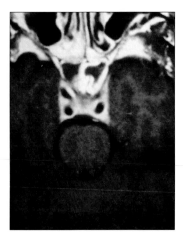

Figure 12.3 MRI or CT neuromaging can be used to diagnose sphenoid sinusitis.

Summary

- Sinusitis is overdiagnosed as a cause of headache.
- Recurrent episodic pain in the sinus areas is more likely to be migrainous with secondary (neurovascular) changes in the sinuses producing the local symptoms.
- Acute sinus disease can clearly cause headache, which can be easily diagnosed by the clinical presentation and which frequently fulfils specific IHS diagnostic criteria. However, the relationship between headache and subacute and chronic sinus disease is unclear. The clinical features of a severe, intractable, new-onset headache that interferes with sleep and is not relieved by simple analgesics should alert the physician to the possibility of sphenoid sinusitis.
- While sphenoid sinusitis is an uncommon cause of headache, it may have significant morbidity and mortality and must be identified early and managed aggressively.

Further reading

Kennedy DW. Overview. *Otolaryngol Head Neck Surg* 1990; 103: 847–54.

Kibblewhite DJ, Cleland J, Mintz DR. Acute sphenoid sinusitis: management strategies. *J Otolaryngol* 1988; 17: 159–63.

Lew D, Southwick FS, Montgomery WW, Weber AL, Baker AS. Sphenoid sinusitis: a review of 30 cases. *N Engl J Med* 1983; 19: 1149–54.

Low DE, Desrosiers M, McSherry J *et al*. A practical guide for the diagnosis and treatment of acute sinusitis. *CMAJ* 1997; 156(6S): 1S–14S.

Saunte C, Soyka D. Headache related to ear, nose, and sinus disorders. In: Olesen J, Tfelt-Hansen P, Welch JMA (eds). *The Headaches*. New York: Raven Press, 1993: 753–7.

Schønsted-Madsen U, Stoksted, P, Christensen, P-H, Koch-Henriksen N. Chronic headache related to nasal obstruction. *J Laryngol Otol* 1986; 100: 165–70.

Williams JW, Simel DL, Roberts L, Samsa GP. Clinical evaluation for sinusitis. *Ann Intern Med* 1992; 117: 705–10.

13 Headache associated with central nervous system infection

Introduction

Patients with central nervous system (CNS) infections may present with headaches that may continue even after adequate treatment. Headaches are associated with a wide range of infections in intracranial and extracranial structures. The International Headache Society system divides infections into intracranial, extracranial, and those that affect the cranium itself as well as associated structures (Table 13.1). The huge array of infectious disorders that produce headache is outside the scope of this chapter (see Further reading). However, in this chapter we highlight selected intracranial infections, including meningitis and encephalitis, Lyme borreliosis, and acquired immunodeficiency syndrome (AIDS), which are relatively common clinical problems.

Meningitis

Meningitis refers to an infectious or inflammatory process of the meninges, which are the membranes that surround the brain and spinal cord. Meningitis is classified according to the pathogen, most commonly viral or bacterial. Other pathogens occur mainly in the setting of primary or secondary immune deficiency states. In the United States, 5–10 cases of acute *bacterial* meningitis occur annually per 100,000 population. Meningitis occurs most frequently in children under 5 years of age. Other predisposing factors are sickle cell disease, alcoholism, and AIDS and other immunocompromised states. *Viral* meningitis occurs mostly in summer in 10.9 cases per 100,000 population. Most cases occur in children and young adults; it is less common after 30 years of age, and the rate is highest in men.

Clinical features

The clinical features of bacterial and viral meningitis are similar, although bacterial meningitis is generally more fulminant. Typically, the headache of bacterial meningitis quickly progresses (at times over minutes) from mild to severe and may

● **Table 13.1** Classification of headaches associated with infection

7	Headaches associated with non-vascular intracranial disorders
	7.3 Intracranial infections
9	Headaches associated with non-cephalic infections
	9.1 Viral infection
	9.2 Bacterial infection
	9.3 Headache related to other infections
11	Headache or facial pain associated with disorders of the cranium, neck, eyes, ears, nose, sinuses, teeth, mouth or other facial or cranial structures

be the first symptom. The headache is usually generalized, sometimes frontal, with bilateral occipital and neck radiation. Pain may radiate down the back and into the extremities, and eye movements are often painful. Patients withdraw from sensory stimulation, avoiding light (photophobia) and sound (phonophobia), and they may have cognitive dysfunction (trouble concentrating and thinking). Nausea, vomiting, and fever with flushing are common. Alteration of consciousness and seizures may occur. Thunderclap headache that increases in severity within minutes may be the first symptom, although young children usually do not complain of headache.

Signs of acute bacterial meningitis include fever, stiff neck (which is worse on flexion than rotation), and alteration of consciousness. Kernig's and Brudzinski's signs are often present. Patients maintain a flexed posture with neck muscles tensed and head extended. Cranial nerve palsies may be present. Infants may present with fever and a bulging fontanelle. The elderly have less prominent headaches than young adults do. Meningitis may include signs that implicate the original site of infection, such as an upper respiratory infection or otitis media. A rash may be present in meningococcal meningitis.

In chronic meningitis, such as tuberculous meningitis, headache and fever may occur in isolation. A chronic headache that increases in severity over weeks to months without fever or other neurological finding is the most common symptom of cryptococcal meningitis. Systemic features, such as fever and myalgias (muscle pains), are variably present. Cognition may be intact or gradually deteriorate. Some chronic meningitides, such as tuberculosis or cryptococcal infection, may produce hydrocephalus with progressive gait ataxia, cognitive decline, or urinary incontinence. Chronic syndromes also occur with brucellar meningitis or Lyme disease.

If a CNS infection is suspected as the cause of headache, lumbar puncture is often the critical diagnostic test. If acute bacterial meningitis is suspected, rapid initiation of therapy may be lifesaving. Lumbar puncture may be performed without imaging if no contraindications or obstacles are present. Contraindications to lumbar puncture without neuroimaging include signs of increased intracranial pressure (papilloedema, coma, anisocoria, fixed pupils), focal neurological signs, suspicion of a CNS mass lesion, a skin infection at the lumbar puncture site, or coagulopathy that cannot be corrected even temporarily. Obstacles include unstable vital signs and the need for ventilatory assistance. When bacterial meningitis is suspected and a mass lesion has been ruled out clinically or by neuroimaging, the cerebrospinal fluid (CSF) should be examined for:

- gram-stain and culture;
- glucose (usually <40 mg/dl or <50% of the blood glucose);
- protein (significantly elevated);
- cell counts (usually >1000 cells/mm^3 with polymorphonuclear predominance);
- elevation of CSF opening pressure; and
- specific bacterial antigen and endotoxin assays.

Blood cultures should be drawn since they are positive in more than 50% of cases of bacterial meningitis. Radiographs of the skull and sinuses may reveal a site of infection or portal of entry into the CNS, although radiography is not routinely used. Magnetic resonance imaging (MRI) may show meningeal enhancement, but it is seldom necessary in typical cases. The peripheral white blood count is likely to be elevated, with a predominance of polymorphonuclear cells and immature forms, supporting the diagnosis of a bacterial process.

A suspected case of meningitis is defined by CSF examination. A microbiological differential diagnosis must be carefully formulated with advice from an infectious disease specialist when chronic meningitis is suspected. Treatment is directed to specific therapy that includes antibiotic, antiviral, or antifungal agents and supportive measures, such as fluids and antipyretics.

Bacterial meningitis

Bacterial meningitis remains a deadly disease for which rapid assessment is essential and can be lifesaving. Bacterial infections present typically with fever, headache, and neck stiffness. The most common agents are listed in Table 13.2. In adults, the most common organisms are *Streptococcus pneumoniae* and *Neisseria meningitidis*. Meningitis due to *Haemophilus influenzae* Type B in children is less common as a result of immunization. However, for immunocompromised patients (those with human immunodeficiency virus [HIV] infection, haematological, and other malignancies or those undergoing chronic immunosuppressive treatment), a search for more unusual pathogens is mandatory. Enteric Gram-negative bacteria need to be considered in newborn infants, patients over 60 years of age, and patients who have had neurosurgery or are immunosuppressed. *Listeria monocytogenes* may also cause meningitis in these groups. Bacterial meningitis may complicate sinusitis, skull fractures, mastoiditis, or local cranial infections and may be a manifestation of a primary infection at any site, such as in osteomyelitis or pneumonia. In a bacterial infection, the CNS has a purulent exudate that is reflected in a highly active CSF, with neutrophils, protein, and a low glucose when compared with a contemporaneous blood glucose level. Once suspected, there should be no delay in treating the

Table 13.2 Common causes of acute bacterial infections in the central nervous system

Haemophilus influenzae

Neisseria meningitidis

Streptococcus pneumoniae

Streptococcus spp. (group B)

Listeria monocytogenes

Escherichia coli

Staphylococcus aureus and S. epidermidis

● **Table 13.3** *Empiric treatment for meningitis*

Age	Common bacterial pathogens	Empirical antimicrobial therapy*
0–4 weeks	*Streptococcus agalactiae, Escherichia coli, Listeria monocytogenes, Kliebsella pneumoniae*	Ampicillin plus cefotaxime, or ampicillin plus aminoglycoside
4–12 weeks	*S. agalactiae, E. coli, L. monocytogenes, Haemophilus influenzae, S. pneumoniae, Neisseria meninigitides*	Ampicillin plus third-generation cephalosporin†
3 months to 18 years	*H. influenzae‡, N. meninigitides, S. pneumoniae*	Third-generation cephalosporin† ± ampicillin§, or ampicillin plus chloramphenicol
18–50 years	*S. pneumoniae, N. meninigitides*	Third-generation cephalosporin† ± ampicillin§
>50 years	*S. pneumoniae, N. meninigitides, L. monocytogenes, aerobic Gram-negative bacilli*	Ampicillin plus third-generation cephalosporin†

*Vancomycin should be added to empirical regimens when highly penicillin- or cephalosporin-resistant pneumococcal meningitis is suspected.

†Cefotaxime or ceftriaxone.

‡Incidence of invasive disease caused by H. influenzae Type B has decreased in countries, such as the United States, in which conjugate vaccines have been introduced.

§Add if meningitis caused by L. monocytogenes is suspected (e.g. in patients with deficiencies in cell-mediated immunity).

infection with antibiotics that cover the pathogens expected in the community or hospital where the infection was acquired (Tables 13.3, 13.4).

Nonbacterial infections

Aseptic meningitis is characterized by severe, rapid-onset headache, fever, malaise, anorexia, phono-phobia, photophobia, and neck rigidity. Consciousness may be altered, although it rarely progresses to obtundation or coma. All patients (except perhaps children) who have aseptic menin-gitis experience a severe, bilateral headache. Generally, non-bacterial intracranial infections follow a more benign clinical course. Many patients who have headache, fever, and neck stiffness are managed with antibiotics, and the diagnosis is questioned when no obvious response occurs. In asep-tic meningitis, CSF examination may reveal:

- CSF cell count (<100 cells/mm^3) with mild pleocytosis usually indicates viral meningitis (early in the course, polymorphonuclear cells may predominate, but this rapidly shifts to lymphocytic pleocytosis);
- CSF pressure is normal or slightly elevated;
- CSF protein is normal or slightly elevated; and
- CSF glucose is normal or slightly reduced.

An excess of lymphocytes, an unremarkable or modestly elevated CSF protein, and a normal ratio of CSF to blood plasma glucose suggest a non-bacterial infection. The peripheral white blood count may be normal or elevated with a normal differential cell count. If the diagnosis is in doubt, antibiotics should be started and the lumbar punc-ture repeated after 12 hours to document the shift from polymorphonuclear cells to mononuclear cells. In some patients, the virus can be isolated from other sites, such as the throat and stool.

Since aseptic meningitis is usually viral, with the enteroviruses (echo, coxsackie, polio), mumps virus, and the arboviruses being the most

● **Table 13.4** *Treatment for common bacterial pathogens*

Micro-organism	Therapy
Haemophilus influenzae Type B	Third-generation cephalosporin*
Neisseria meninigitides	Penicillin G or ampicillin or third-generation cephalosporin*
Streptococcus pneumoniae	Vancomycin plus third-generation cephalosporin*†
Listeria monocytogenes	Ampicillin or penicillin G‡
Streptococcus agalactiae	Ampicillin or penicillin G‡
Escherichia coli	Third-generation cephalosporin*

*Cefotaxime or ceftriaxone.

†Addition of rifampicin may be considered.

‡Addition of aminoglycoside should be considered.

common causative organisms (Table 13.5), CSF should be analysed for viral antigens and incubated for viral culture. Virus prevalence is often geographical and seasonal, and the causative virus is isolated in only 11–12% of patients. Other conditions that resemble aseptic meningitis include fungal meningitis, parameningeal infections, non-infectious conditions (malignant meningitis, sarcoidosis, or chemical meningitis from spinal anaesthesia, myelography, or intrathecal medications), and bacterial agents that are difficult to culture, such as those causing syphilis (*Treponema palladium*), tuberculosis (*Mycobacterium tuberculosis*), and Lyme disease (*Borrelia burgdorferi*).

Lyme disease

Neuroborreliosis or Lyme disease of the nervous system produces a pleomorphic clinical picture that may include lymphocytis, meningitis with or without cranial nerve lesions, encephalomyelitis, encephalopathy, and radiculopathy and neuropathy of either cranial or peripheral nerves. Lyme disease is a multisystem infection caused by the spirochete *B. burgdorferi*. Early in this tick-borne illness, patients may have a characteristic cutaneous lesion, erythema migrans (Figure 13.1). Some patients develop disseminated and then chronic infections with prominent neurological, rheumatological, and cardiac

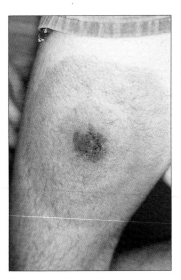

● *Figure 13.1 Rash of Lyme disease (Erythema Chronicum Migrans).*

● **Table 13.5** *Common viral pathogens in meningitis*

Enterovirus	Epstein–Barr virus
Coxsackie A and B	Rubella
Cytomegalovirus	Mumps
Herpes simplex	Adenovirus
Herpes zoster	Human immunodeficiency virus

manifestations. During erythema migrans, headache occurs in 38–54% of patients and presents few diagnostic challenges.

Headache as the most prominent manifestation of Lyme borreliosis

Several authors have recommended a work-up for Lyme borreliosis when headaches are atypical, especially if the onset is subacute. Occasionally, headache is the most prominent neurological manifestation of CNS Lyme disease. Several reports describe patients with rapidly progressive chronic headache who were eventually evaluated for Lyme disease. Several patients have had positive CSF Lyme antibody indices, which provide strong evidence for CNS infection with *B. burgdorferi*. In these cases, the headaches completely resolved after treatment with ceftriaxone.

Laboratory tests

We summarize here some selected tests that may be helpful to diagnose patients with headache and suspected Lyme disease – serological tests (enzyme-linked immunosorbent assay [ELISA]) for Lyme demonstrate possible exposure, not current infection. Since 5–10% of asymptomatic individuals in endemic areas have positive serology, most positive serological tests in otherwise asymptomatic headache patients will be false positives. The Western blot test characterizes the specific *B. burgdorferi* antigens and serves primarily to confirm a positive ELISA or to identify a false positive result.

Demonstrating antibody production within the CNS relies on the ratio of antibody in CSF to antibody in serum. These procedures are quite valid and may even be positive when peripheral serological tests are negative. In addition, culture and polymerase chain reaction (PCR) can be carried out. These are highly specific, but are not always positive.

Preliminary recommendations

- Routine testing for Lyme disease is not recommended for patients who present with headache. The false-positive tests would most likely lead to inappropriate evaluation or treatment.
- If a headache is accompanied by apparent systemic or neurological manifestations suggestive of Lyme disease, serum antibody testing by ELISA is suggested.
- For patients with atypical headaches (rapid increase to near-daily headaches, unusual associated symptoms, or poor response to treatment), serological testing for Lyme disease should be considered. A suspected false-positive ELISA should be confirmed by a Western blot for *Borrelia*-specific antigens.
- Patients with headache as the sole neurological manifestation and a positive ELISA and Western blot should be treated with oral doxycycline 100 mg by mouth, twice daily for 3 or 4 weeks. If the headache does not remit, lumbar puncture should be considered.
- For patients with headache and evidence of Lyme-related neurological disorders or dysfunction (such as encephalopathy, cognitive defects, focal deficits), neuroimaging and lumbar puncture for cell count, protein glucose, and Lyme antibody index should be carried out. If CNS disease is present, intravenous therapy should be considered and appropriate neurological referral sought.

Encephalitis

Encephalitis is an infection that involves the brain parenchyma and is usually caused by a virus (Table 13.6). In the United States, 7.4 per 100,000 population have viral encephalitis annually, mostly in the summer and early autumn, with the incidence highest in infants. Men are affected more often than women. Encephalitis is characterized by headache, fever, alteration of consciousness,

● **Table 13.6** Common causes of encephalitis

Mumps	Toxoplasmosis
Arbovirus	Epstein–Barr virus
Herpes simplex	Adenovirus
Herpes zoster	

focal neurological deficit, seizures (usually focal), and, sometimes, meningeal signs. Headache alone may be the initial manifestation of encephalitis. A prodrome of less severe but constant headache associated with malaise, mild fever, and myalgia may precede the onset of the neurological deficit by several days. Herpes simplex virus encephalitis typically has no identifiable systemic prodrome, but the patient may present with behavioural changes or memory disturbance.

Encephalitis is marked clinically by impaired cognition and sometimes by distinct focal neurological clinical syndromes. Patients usually have headache, fever, and stiff neck, although headache and impaired consciousness may be the only clinical manifestation. The cerebral picture may be predated by a prodrome of feeling generally unwell, with fever, malaise, or myalgia for up to a week prior to the more acute presentation. While some encephalitides are clinically mild, some, like herpes simplex, can be devastating. The infection very often involves the temporal cortex bilaterally and is almost invariably accompanied by an abnormal electroencephalogram. Patients with suspected herpes simplex encephalitis require early treatment with antiviral agents in adequate doses. In immunosuppressed patients, certain pathogens, such as toxoplasmosis, cryptococcoses, and cytomegalovirus, are more common and must be actively sought out.

Special problems

Acquired immunodeficiency syndrome

One of the most challenging conditions that predisposes to intracranial infection, HIV also produces headache. Headache can occur in the acute phase of HIV, as part of HIV meningitis or encephalitis, or with the secondary infections that are frequently seen in these patients. Particularly common is toxoplasmosis, which is often seen as multiple contrast-enhancing lesions on computed tomography. Meningitis in AIDS can involve any of the common pathogens, but types rarer in a general Western population often occur in AIDS patients. Cryptococcal infection is common and relatively easily diagnosed by means of CSF examination with India ink stain and cryptococcal antigen testing. Similarly, tuberculous meningitis is often seen in AIDS patients and must be sought diligently by means of CSF examination using PCR techniques.

Brain abscess

Signs and symptoms of brain abscess depend on the location of the abscess and the amount of mass effect it produces. Although headache is the most common presenting symptom, the patient may present with a seizure. Focal neurological signs and altered mental status are common. Signs of an antecedent infection, such as otitis media, sinusitis, a dental infection, or endocarditis, may be present. Fever and leucocytosis are less likely to be present, but nausea and vomiting often begin a week after headache onset. These symptoms may result from increased intracranial pressure, although less than half the patients have papilloedema at presentation. With a cerebellar abscess, the headache is often suboccipital with associated cervical pain and rigidity.

Brain abscess occurs in approximately 1 per 100,000 population annually, with peak incidence in childhood and after 60 years of age. Three times more common in men than in women, the risk factors include neurosurgery, penetrating brain trauma, and, particularly in children, otitis media. Aerobic or anaerobic bacteria cause brain abscess, and they often contain multiple organisms that come from the source of the infection. Examples include *Staphylococcus aureus* and *Bacteroides* that occur with otitis media, mastoiditis, or that occur with open head trauma or sinusitis, and streptococci, staphylococci, or Gram-negative rods that occur with open head trauma or neurosurgery. Overall, there is a high incidence of *S. milleri* isolated from brain abscesses of all causes.

Neuroimaging is the diagnostic procedure of choice for brain abscesses. The CT scan shows a central area of decreased attenuation surrounded by a ring of intense contrast enhancement, which may then be surrounded by oedema. The presence of gas within the lesion supports the diagnosis. Although MRI may be superior to CT in its ability to detect early cerebritis, oedema, minor haemorrhage, and disruption of the blood–brain barrier, it is sometimes not available. Since brain tumour, cerebral infarct, and radiation necrosis may appear identical to abscess on CT scan, diagnostic (and therapeutic) neurosurgical intervention is often necessary. However, the growing availability of MRI makes *diagnostic* intervention less necessary.

The abscess should be incised, drained, and sent for bacterial culture and biopsy. Routine blood tests rarely help in diagnosis since the peripheral white blood count is usually normal or only slightly elevated. Blood cultures should be drawn if endocarditis is suspected.

Headache treatment

The headache of intracranial infection should resolve with treatment of the underlying condition. Until the infection has cleared, non-opioid analgesics may be used or, if severe, opioids may be used, bearing in mind that they may obscure some aspects of the neurological examination (e.g. level of consciousness and pupil size). If the headache persists long after the infection and its complications have resolved, the patient may require evaluation and treatment of chronic headache. These headaches behave as post-traumatic headaches (*see* Chapter 10). In general terms, the infection seems to act as a 'trauma' and the course and treatment of the headache follows that of headache after head injury.

Summary

- Headache that increases in severity within minutes may be the first symptom of acute bacterial meningitis. Such headache is less prominent in children.
- Most patients with aseptic meningitis experience a headache that is usually bilateral and often severe. Such headache is less prominent in children and in the elderly.
- Almost half of patients with Lyme disease have headache during erythema migrans; some patients present with chronic tension-type headache as the most prominent neurological symptom of CNS Lyme disease or meningitis or encephalitis.
- Patients with encephalitis may exhibit thunderclap headache alone or accompanied by fever, alteration of consciousness, focal neurological deficit, or seizures.
- AIDS patients experience headache in the acute phase of the infection, as part of HIV meningitis or encephalitis, and in the setting of secondary infections (toxoplasmosis or progressive multifocal leukoencephalopathy) or chronic meningitis (cryptococcal meningitis).
- Headache is the most common presenting symptom in the patient with a brain abscess, although the patient may also present with seizure.
- A small number of patients experience chronic headaches even after the infection is successfully treated; these patients require specialist review.

Further reading

Bharucha NE, Bhaba SK, Bharucha EP. Infections of the nervous system. B viral infections. In: Bradley WG, Daroff RB, Fenichel GM, Marsden CE (eds). *Neurology in Clinical Practice*. Stoneham: Butterworth-Heinemann, 1991: 1085–97.

Fishman RA. *Cerebrospinal Fluid in Diseases of the Nervous System*, 2nd edn. Philadelphia: WB Saunders, 1992.

Isenberg H. Bacterial meningitis: signs and symptoms. *Antiobiot Chemother* 1992; 45: 79–95.

Kaplan K. Brain abscess. *Med Clin North Am* 1985; 69(2): 345–60.

Lakeman FD, Koga J, Whitley RJ. Detection of antigen to Herpes simplex virus in cerebrospinal fluid from patients with Herpes simplex encephalitis. *J. Infect Dis* 1987; 155(6): 1172–8.

Oliver LG, Harwood-Nuss AL. Bacterial meningitis in infants and children: a review. *J Emerg Med* 1993; 11: 555–64.

Silberstein SD. Headache associated with meningitis, encephalitis, and brain abscess. *Neurobase* La Jolla: Arbar, 1997.

Tunkel AR, Scheld MW. Acute bacterial meningitis. *Lancet* 1995; 346: 1675–80; *Medical Letter* 1996; 38: 25.

Wood M, Anderson M (eds). *Neurological Infections*. WB Saunders, 1988.

14 Pregnancy, breastfeeding, and headache

Pregnancy

Every type of headache can occur in the pregnant patient, and while a certain emphasis is necessary, the general rules about headache developed in earlier chapters still apply. Migraine, tension-type headache, and other primary headaches occur during pregnancy, as do the conditions that mimic them – vasculitis, brain tumour, and occipital arteriovenous malformation (AVM). Some women experience their first migraine during pregnancy; however, 60–70% of migraineurs experience improvement or cessation of their headaches during pregnancy. For a smaller group of migraineurs, headache either worsens, particularly in the first trimester, or remains unchanged. The true incidence of migraine in pregnancy is unknown. Other headache disorders occur during pregnancy, including sinusitis, meningitis, idiopathic intracranial hypertension, and subarachnoid haemorrhage (SAH), which require neuroimaging or lumbar puncture to diagnose them.

The headache-producing disorders that occur more frequently or exclusively during pregnancy include stroke, cerebral venous thrombosis, eclampsia, SAH, pituitary tumour, and choriocarcinoma (Table 14.1). Diagnostic tests that expose the fetus to the least risk should be used to exclude organic causes of headache, confirm the diagnosis, and establish a baseline before treatment.

● **Table 14.1** Headache disorders and pregnancy

Less common	As common	More common
Migraine	Idiopathic intracranial hypertension	Stroke
Menstrual headache	Tension-type headache	Cerebral venous thrombosis
	Sinusitis	Eclampsia
	Meningitis	Subarachnoid haemorrhage
	Vasculitis	Pituitary tumour
	Brain tumour	Choriocarcinoma

Most drugs are probably not teratogenic, but not enough is known about drug effects during pregnancy. While medication use should be limited, it is not absolutely contraindicated in pregnancy. In migraine, the risk of status migrainosus may be greater than the potential risk of the medication used to treat the pregnant patient. While non-pharmacological treatment is the ideal solution, analgesics, such as paracetamol (acetaminophen), and narcotics can be used on a limited basis. Preventive therapy is a last resort.

Neurodiagnostic testing: radiology

Radiation's effect on the developing fetus is a major concern. Unless an aneurysm, an AVM, or vasculitis is suspected, there is little reason to perform angiography in a pregnant (or non-pregnant) patient with a normal neurological examination, a normal computed tomography (CT) or magnetic resonance imaging (MRI), and a history consistent with a benign primary headache disorder. The potential risk of MRI in pregnancy is still unclear. Magnetic resonance magnets induce an electric field and raise the core temperature by less than 1°C. High body temperature may increase the incidence of neural tube defects, and other effects of MRI are not known. Gadolinium, a contrast agent used with MRI, crosses the placental barrier and is excreted through the fetal kidneys. Although no ill effects have been demonstrated, gadolinium injection should be avoided, as should CT contrast media.

Head CT, which is relatively safe during pregnancy, is the study of choice for head trauma and possible non-traumatic subarachnoid, subdural, or intraparenchymal haemorrhage. For all other non-traumatic or non-haemorrhagic craniospinal pathology, MRI is preferred. Magnetic resonance angiography is used first to evaluate any suspected vascular pathology. If cranial angiography is needed, the patient should be referred to a neurologist.

Potential indications for CT or MRI in headache investigation during pregnancy include:

- first or worst headache of the patient's life, particularly one with abrupt onset (thunderclap headache);
- marked change in frequency, severity, or clinical features of the headache attack;
- abnormal neurological examination;
- new daily persistent headache;
- neurological symptoms that do not meet the criteria of migraine with typical aura;
- persistent neurological defects;
- an orbital or skull bruit suggestive of AVM; and
- new comorbid partial (focal) seizures.

In each case, the physician must judge the risk of not diagnosing the condition against minor radiation risk (Table 14.2).

Table 14.2 Guidelines for neuroimaging the patient who is or may be pregnant

- Determine the necessity and the potential risks of the procedure
- If possible, perform the examination during the first 10 days postmenses, or if the patient is pregnant, delay the examination until the third trimester or preferably postpartum
- Pick the procedure with the highest accuracy balanced by the lowest radiation
- Use MRI if possible
- Avoid direct exposure to the abdomen and pelvis
- Avoid contrast agents
- Do not avoid radiological testing purely for the sake of the pregnancy
- If significant exposure is incurred by a pregnant patient, consult a radiation biologist
- Consent forms are neither required nor recommended

Adapted from Schwartz, 1994.

Migraine and Pregnancy

Mechanisms

The relief that many pregnant migraineurs experience may be the result of rising or sustained high oestrogen levels. However, this mechanism cannot explain the new-onset or worsened migraine that sometimes occurs. The rapid fall of oestrogen levels may be responsible for menstrual and postpartum migraine – women with a prior history of migraine are more likely to have migraine during the postpartum period. Migraine relief during pregnancy does not depend on adequate 'protective' levels of progesterone.

Study series

Several groups have studied the incidence and course of migraine during menstruation and pregnancy – the findings are summarized in Tables 14.3 and 14.4. In general, most women experience migraine improvement with pregnancy, but women who have menstrual migraine seem to do best.

Outcome of pregnancy in migraineurs

The incidence of miscarriage, toxaemia, congenital anomalies, or stillbirths does not increase in migraineurs when compared with national averages or controls.

Postnatal migraine

Postnatal headache (PNH) occurs in about 39% of women (and in 58% of those women with a history of migraine), most frequently on days 3–6 postpartum. Although PNH is associated with a personal or family history of migraine, it is less severe than the patient's typical headache, and is bifrontal and prolonged, with photophobia, nausea, and anorexia. Migraine often recurs or begins in the postpartum period.

Treatment
Risk of drug treatment

Of the 3000 drugs tested by the United States Food and Drug Administration (FDA), only 20 are known human teratogens (Table 14.5). Of women who are pregnant, 67% take drugs, 50% in the first trimester. However, not enough is known about birth-defect risks. Most drugs cross the placenta and have the potential to affect the fetus adversely. Although studies have not established the safety of any medication during pregnancy, some drugs are believed to be relatively safe (see Tables 14.6–14.10). Fetal death, teratogenicity, fetal growth abnormalities, perinatal effects, postnatal developmental abnormalities, delayed oncogenesis, and functional and behavioural changes can result from drugs or other agents (Table 14.5). According to the Perinatal Collaborative Project, which is a prospective and concurrent epidemiological study

Table 14.3 *Migraine and pregnancy*

Parameter	Lance and Anthony (1966)	Callaghan (1968)	Somerville (1970)	Bousser et al. (1990)	Granella et al. (1993)	Rasmussen (1993)	Chen and Leviton (1994)	Maggioni et al. (1995)
Women studied		200	200	703	1300	975	55,000	428
History of migraine and pregnancies	120	41	38	116	943	80	484	80
Number of pregnancies	252	200	200	147	943		484	?
New migraine during pregnancy	0	33/41 (80%)	7/38 (18%)	16/147 (11%)	12 (1.3%)	?	0	1/428
New migraine postpartum				?	42 (4.5%)	?	0	?
Prior migraine	252	8	31	131	571	80	484	91
Prior migraine improved	145/252 (58%)	4 (50%)	24/31 (77%)	102/131 (78%)	384/571 (67.3%)	48%	382/484 (79%)	80%
Prior migraine unchanged or worsened	107/252 (42%)	3 (38%)	7/31 (23%)	29/131 (22%)	187/571 (32.7%)	52%	102/484 (21%)	20%
Type series	R, H	R, H	R, H	R, O	R, H	R, POP	P, O	R, H

H = headache or neurological; P = prospective; R = retrospective; POP = population base

Table 14.4 *Menstrual migraine and migraine improvement with pregnancy*

Menstrual/non-menstrual	Lance (1966)	Bousser et al. (1990)
Menstrual		
Disappeared or improved	64%	86%
Worsened	36%	7%
Non-menstrual		
Disappeared or improved	48%	60%
Worsened	52%	15%

Table 14.5 *Definitions and drug effects*

Spontaneous abortion	Death of the conceptus. Most due to chromosomal abnormality.
Embryotoxicity	The ability of drugs to kill the developing embryo.
Congenital anomalies	Deviation from normal morphology or function.
Teratogenicity	The ability of an exogenous agent to produce a permanent abnormality of structure or function in an organism exposed during embryogenesis or fetal life.
Fetal effects	Growth retardation, abnormal histogenesis (also congenital abnormalities and fetal death). These are main outcome of fetal drug toxicity during the second and third trimesters of pregnancy.
Perinatal effects	Effects on uterine contraction, neonatal withdrawal, or haemostasis.
Postnatal effects	Drugs may have delayed long-term effects: delayed oncogenesis and functional and behavioural abnormalities.

of more than 50,000 pregnancies, many drugs have little or no human teratogenic risk.

Drug risk categories

The FDA lists five categories of labels for drug use in pregnancy (Table 14.6). These categories provide therapeutic guidance, weighing the risks and benefits of each drug. An alternative rating system is TERIS, an automated teratogen information resource designed to assess the teratogenic risk to the fetus from a drug exposure; it is used by more than 900 specialized centres throughout the world. In TERIS, ratings for each drug or agent are based on a consensus of expert opinion and the literature (Table 14.7).

● **Table 14.6** FDA risk categories

Category A	Controlled human studies show no risk
Category B	No evidence of risk in humans, but there are no controlled human studies
Category C	Risk to humans has not been ruled out
Category D	Positive evidence of risk to humans from human and/or animal studies
Category X	Contraindicated in pregnancy.

● **Table 14.7** TERIS risk rating

- Undetermined (C)
- None (A)
- None–minimal (A)
- Minimal (B)
- Minimal–small (D)
- High (X)

Equivalent FDA ratings in parentheses.

● **Table 14.8** Some therapeutic medications

Drug class		Fetal risk	
		FDA[*]	**TERIS**
Simple analgesics	Aspirin	C (D)	None–minimal
	Acetaminophen	B	None
	Caffeine	B	None–minimal
NSAIDs	Ibuprofen	B (D)	None–minimal
	Indomethacin	B (D)	None
	Naproxen	B (D)	Undetermined
Opioids	Butorphanol	C (D)	None–minimal
	Codeine	C (D)	None–minimal
	Pethidine (meperidine)	B (D)	None–minimal
	Methadone	B (D)	None–minimal
	Morphine	B (D)	None–minimal
	Dextropropoxyphene (propoxyphene)	C (D)	None–minimal
Ergots Serotonin agonists	Ergotamine	X	Minimal
	Dihydroergotamine	X	Undetermined
	Sumatriptan	C	Undetermined
	Eletriptan	C	None–minimal
	Naratriptan	C	None–minimal
	Rizatriptan	C	None–minimal
	Zolmitriptan	C	None–minimal
Corticosteroids	Dexamethasone	C	None–minimal
	Prednisone	B	None–minimal
Barbiturates	Butalbital	C (D)	None–minimal
	Phenobarbital	D	None–minimal
Benzodiazepam	Chlordiazepoxide	D	None–minimal
	Clonazepam	D	Uncertain
	Diazepam	D	None–minimal

[*]Risk factor if used at end of third trimester given in parentheses.

● **Table 14.9** Neuroleptics and antiemetics

Drug class		Fetal risk	
		FDA	**TERIS**
Antihistamines	Cyclizine	B	Undetermined
	Cyproheptadine	B	Undetermined
	Dimenhydrinate	B	None–minimal
	Meclozine	B	None–minimal
Neuroleptics	Phenothiazines		
	Chlorpromazine	C	None–minimal
	Prochlorperazine	C	None
	Butyrophenones	C	None–minimal
	Haloperidol		
	Metoclopramide	B	None–minimal
Other	Emetrol	B	Unknown
	Doxylamine succinate	–	None
	Vitamin B_6 (pyridoxine)	B	None

A woman's risk of having a child with a neural tube defect is associated with early pregnancy red cell folate levels in a continuous dose–response relationship. In one small study, women with epilepsy who were taking phenytoin needed 1 mg of folate supplement a day to maintain a normal serum level. The current guidelines suggest increasing folic acid intake by 4 mg, which would result in a 48% reduction in neural tube defects. Supplementing this by fortifying food with folate would benefit all women.

Headache treatment

The major concern in managing the pregnant migraine patient is the effect of both headache and migraine medication on the fetus. The possible risk to the fetus requires that medication use should be limited. However, medication is not contraindicated during pregnancy. Since migraine usually improves after the first trimester, many women can manage their headaches, with reassurance about the improvement and the use of non-pharmacological means, such as ice, massage, and biofeedback. Some women, however, continue to have severe, intractable headaches, sometimes with nausea, vomiting, and dehydration. These manifestations may pose a risk to the fetus that is greater than the potential risk from taking

Table 14.10 *Guidelines for prophylactic treatment*

Drug class	Dose	Fetal risk	
		FDA	**TERIS**
β-blockers			
Atenolol	50–120 mg/day	C	Undetermined
Metoprolol	50–100 mg/day	B	Undetermined
Nadolol	40–240 mg/day	C	Undetermined
Propranolol	40–320 mg/day	C	Undetermined
Timolol	10–30 mg/day	C	Undetermined
Antidepressants			
Tricyclics			
Amitriptyline	10–250 mg/day	D	None–minimal
Doxepin	10–150–mg/day	C	Undetermined
Nortriptyline HCl	10–100 mg/day	D	Undetermined
Protriptyline	5–60 mg/day	C	Undetermined
SSRIs			
Fluoxetine	10–80 mg/day	B	None
Paroxetine	10–50 mg/day	C	Undetermined
Sertraline	25–200 mg/day	B	Unknown
Calcium-channel blockers			
Verapamil	240–720 mg/day	C	Undetermined
Nifedipine	30–180 mg/day	C	Undetermined
Diltiazem	120–360 mg/day	C	Undetermined
Serotonin agonists			
Methysergide	2–8 mg/day in divided doses up to 14 mg/day	D	Undetermined
Methylergo-novine maleate	0.2–0.4 mg q6h	C	Undetermined
Pizotifen	1–6 mg/day	C	Undetermined
Anticonvulsants			
Divalproex sodium	500–3000 mg/day	D	Small–moderate

medications. Women who are not pregnant, but who are attempting to become pregnant or who are not using adequate birth control, need guidance. The principles are the same as for pregnant women with the caveat that menstrual migraine (which implies that the patient is not yet pregnant) can be treated more aggressively.

Rest, reassurance, and ice packs are treatments that can be used to reduce the severity and duration of symptoms in an acute headache attack (Tables 14.8 and 14.9). For headaches that do not respond to non-pharmacological treatment, symptomatic drugs are indicated. The non-steroidal anti-inflammatory drugs (NSAIDs), paracetamol (alone or with codeine), codeine alone, or other opioids can be used during pregnancy. Aspirin in low intermittent doses is not a significant teratogenic risk, although large doses, especially if given near term, may cause maternal and fetal bleeding. Aspirin should probably not be given unless there is a definite therapeutic need for it other than headache. Barbiturate and benzodiazepine use should be limited. Ergotamine, dihydroergotamine, and the triptans (sumatriptan, rizatriptan, naratriptan, eletriptan and zolmitriptan) should be avoided.

The symptoms that are often associated with migraine, such as nausea and vomiting, can be as disabling as the headache pain, and some medications that are used to treat migraine may even produce nausea. Metoclopramide is helpful to decrease the gastric atony that occurs with migraine and to enhance the absorption of co-administered medications. Mild nausea can be treated with phosphorylated carbohydrate solution (emetrol) or doxylamine succinate and vitamin B_6 (pyridoxine). More severe nausea may require injections or suppositories. Trimethobenzamide, chlorpromazine, prochlorperazine, and promethazine are available orally, parenterally, and by suppository, and can all be used safely. Corticosteroids can be utilized occasionally. Some physicians prefer prednisone to dexamethasone (which crosses the placenta more readily).

Severe, acute attacks of migraine should be treated aggressively. We start intravenous fluids for hydration and then use prochlorperazine 10 mg intravenously to control nausea and head pain. This combination can be supplemented with intravenous opioids or intravenous corticosteroids for an extremely effective way to handle status migrainosus during pregnancy.

Preventive treatment

Increased frequency and severity of migraine with nausea and vomiting may justify the use of daily preventive medication. This option should be a last resort, to be used only with the consent of the patient and her partner after the risks have been explained to them. The physician can consider prophylaxis when patients experience at least three or four prolonged, severe attacks per month that are incapacitating or unresponsive to symptomatic therapy and that may result in dehydration and fetal distress. Beta-adrenergic blockers, such as propranolol, have been used under these circumstances, although adverse effects including intrauterine growth retardation have been reported. If the migraine is so severe that drug treatment is essential, the patient should be told of the risks posed by all the drugs that are used (Table 14.10). If the patient has a coexistent illness that requires treatment, the physician should pick one drug that will treat both disorders. For example, propranolol can be used to treat hypertension and migraine, while fluoxetine can be used to treat comorbid depression.

Drug exposure

If a woman becomes pregnant while taking a drug or inadvertently takes a drug while pregnant, it is important to determine the dose, timing, and duration of the exposure(s). The physician should ascertain the patient's past and present health, and the presence of mental retardation or chromosomal abnormalities in the family. Using a reliable source, such as TERIS, determine if the drug is a known teratogen (although this is not possible for many drugs). If the drug is teratogenic or its risk is not known and gestational age is determined by ultrasound, the physician should determine whether exposure to the drug occurred during embryogenesis. If so, then high-resolution ultrasound can determine whether damage has occurred to specific fetal organ systems or structures. If the high-resolution ultrasound is normal, it is reasonable to reassure the patient that the gross fetal structure is normal (within 90% sensitivity of the study). However, fetal ultrasound cannot exclude minor anomalies or guarantee the birth of a normal child. Delayed development, including cognitive development, is a potential risk, especially for children born to a woman who has epilepsy, that cannot be predicted or diagnosed prenatally. The physician should discuss this with the mother and her partner; in uncertain cases, prenatal counselling may be helpful.

Breast-feeding

Many drugs can be detected in breast milk at levels that are not of clinical significance to the infant – the concentration of drug in breast milk

● **Table 14.11** *Drug categories and breast-feeding*

- Contraindicated
- Require temporary cessation of breast feeding
- Effects unknown but may be of concern
- Use with caution
- Usually compatible

From American Academy of Pediatrics on Drugs, 1994.

● **Table 14.12** *Prescribing guidelines and breast-feeding*

- Is the drug necessary?
- Use the safest drug (e.g. paracetamol instead of aspirin).
- If there is a possibility that a drug may present a risk to the infant (e.g. phenytoin, phenobarbital), consider measuring the blood level in the nursing infant.
- Drug exposure to the nursing infant may by minimized by having the mother take the medication just after completing a breastfeeding.

From American Academy of Pediatrics on Drugs, 1994.

is a variable fraction of the maternal blood level. The infant dose is usually 1–2% of the maternal dose, which is usually trivial. However, any exposure to a toxin or potential allergen should be avoided.

Classification of drugs used during lactation

The American Academy of Pediatrics Committee on Drugs reviewed drugs taken by lactating women and categorized them, as shown in Table 14.11. When prescribing drugs to lactating women, the guidelines in Table 14.12 should be followed.

The migraineur who breast-feeds should avoid bromocriptine, ergotamine, and lithium, and should use with caution the triptans, benzodiazepines, antidepressants, and neuroleptics. Paracetamol is compatible with breastfeeding and is preferred to aspirin (Tables 14.13–14.15). Moderate caffeine use is compatible with breastfeeding, but caffeine accumulation can occur in infants whose mothers use excessive amounts. Opioid use is compatible with breastfeeding. Phenobarbital has caused sedation in some nursing infants and should be given with caution to nursing mothers.

● **Table 14.13** *Drugs and breast-feeding*

Drug class		Breast-feeding
Simple analgesics	Aspirin	Caution*
	Paracetamol	Compatible
	Caffeine	Compatible
	NSAIDs	Compatible
Opioids		Compatible
Barbiturates		Caution**
Benzodiazepam		Concern***
Antihistamines	Cyproheptadine	Contraindicated
Neuroleptics	Phenothiazines	
	Chlorpromazine	Concern
	Prochlorperazine	Compatible
	Metoclopramide	Concern

* Metabolic acidosis, platelet function abnormality.
** Sedation.
*** Effects unknown but of concern.
From American Academy of Pediatrics Committee on Drugs, 1994.

● **Table 14.14** *Drugs and breast-feeding*

Ergot/serotonin agonists	Breast-feeding
Ergotamine	Contraindicated
Dihydroergotamine	Contraindicated
Methylergonovine maleate	Caution
Methysergide	Caution
Sumatriptan	Caution

From American Academy of Pediatrics Committee on Drugs, 1994.

● **Table 14.15** *Drugs and breast-feeding*

Drug class		Breast-feeding
Antihypertensives	Beta-blockers	Compatible
	Adrenergic blockers	Compatible
	Calcium-channel blockers	Compatible
Antidepressants	Tricyclic antidepressants	Concern
	Selective serotonin reuptake inhibitors	Caution
Other drugs	Carbamazepine	Compatible
	Valproic acid	Compatible
	Corticosteroids	Compatible
	Bromocriptine	Contraindicated

From American Academy of Pediatrics Committee on Drugs, 1994.

Summary

- Some women experience their first migraine during pregnancy. The headaches of migraineurs during pregnancy may change in frequency or severity.
- Tension-type and other primary headaches occur during pregnancy, as do the conditions that mimic them: vasculitis, brain tumour, occipital AVM, sinusitis, meningitis, idiopathic intracranial hypertension, and subarachnoid haemorrhage.
- Incidence of miscarriage, toxaemia, congenital anomalies, or stillbirth does not increase in migraineurs when compared with national averages or controls.
- To the extent possible, treating patients with non-pharmacological means is preferred over medication because of possible risk of injury to the fetus.
- The physician should prescribe a headache drug for a lactating mother only when absolutely necessary, and should use the safest drug with the least exposure to the nursing infant.

Further reading

American Academy of Pediatrics Committee on Drugs. The transfer of drugs and update other chemicals into human milk. *Pediatrics* 1994: 93: 137–50.

Biggs GG, Freeman RK, Yaffe SJ (eds). *Drugs in Pregnancy and Lactation*, 4th edn. Baltimore: Williams & Wilkins, 1994.

Blake DA, Niebyl JR. Requirements and limitations in reproductive and teratogenic risk assessment. In: Niebyl JR (ed.) *Drug Use in Pregnancy,* 2nd edn. Philadelphia: Lea & Febiger 1988: 1–9.

Bousser MG, Ratinahirana H, Darbois X. Migraine and pregnancy: a prospective study in 703 women after delivery. *Abstracts Neurol* 1990; 40(1): 437.

Callaghan N. The migraine syndrome in pregnancy. *Neurology* 1968; 18: 197–201.

Chen TC, Leviton A. Headache recurrence in pregnant women with migraine. *Headache* 1994; 34: 107–10.

Friedman, JM, Polifka JE (eds). *Teratogenic Effects of Drugs: a Resource for Clinicians (TERIS)*. Baltimore: Johns Hopkins University Press, 1994.

Gilstrap LC III, Little BB (eds). *Drugs and Pregnancy.* Elsevier: New York, 1992: 23–9.

Granella F, Sances G, Zanferrari C *et al*. Migraine without aura and reproductive life events: a clinical epidemiologic study in 1300 women. *Headache* 1993; 33: 385–9.

Lance JW, Anthony M. Some clinical aspects of migraine. *Arch Neurol* 1966; 15: 356–61.

Maggioni F, Alessi C, Maggino T *et al*. Primary headaches and pregnancy (abstr). *Cephalalgia* 1995; 15: 54.

Rasmussen BK. Migraine and tension-type headache in a general population: precipitating factors, female hormones, sleep pattern, and relation to lifestyle. *Pain* 1993; 53: 65–72.

Schwartz RB. Neurodiagnostic imaging of the pregnant patient. In: Devinsky O, Feldmann E, Hainline B (eds). *Neurologic Complications of Pregnancy*. New York: Raven Press, 1994: 243–8.

Shepard TH. *Catalog of Teratogenic Agents*, 8th edn. Baltimore: Johns Hopkins University Press, 1973.

Somerville BW. A study of migraine in pregnancy. *Neurology* 1972; 22: 824–8.

15 Geriatric headache

Introduction

Headache prevalence varies with age. Although less common than in the young, headache remains a significant problem in the elderly, with 10% of women and 5% of men reporting severe headaches at 70 years of age. Headache aetiology also varies with age as the incidence of primary headache dramatically declines while the incidence of secondary headache disorders, such as mass lesions and temporal arteritis, increases with increasing age. Some secondary headache disorders, such as giant cell arteritis (GCA), occur almost exclusively in the elderly (Table 15.1). At least one primary headache disorder – the hypnic headache syndrome – is much more common in the elderly. Older patients are also more likely to have comorbid disease. Thus, age is an important factor in the diagnosis and treatment of headache disorders

Table 15.2 summarizes the major causes of headaches that begin late in life. After 65 years of age, headache is more likely to result from serious conditions, systemic illnesses, or medications. Mass lesions and GCA (temporal arteritis) have devastating, but often avoidable, consequences. When older patients present with headache, a full evaluation is indicated to identify or exclude secondary headaches. After 50 years of age, patients with a new onset or new type of headache usually require a neuroimaging procedure (computed tomography or magnetic resonance imaging [MRI]) and an erythrocyte sedimentation rate (ESR) as part of the initial work-up to identify or rule out structural lesions and GCA. After excluding secondary causes, the physician should identify and treat the primary headache (migraine, cluster, and tension-type headache [TTH]) that can begin or recur in the elderly and may present in unusual ways.

In this chapter the major secondary headache disorders in the elderly are discussed. In addition, the section on primary headache disorders emphasizes the diagnostic and treatment dilemmas encountered in elderly patients.

Secondary headache disorders

Mass lesions

Primary and metastatic brain tumours and subdural haematomas (SDH) occur with increased frequency in the elderly. The most frequent primary brain tumours are gliomas, pituitary adenomas, and meningiomas (especially common in

Table 15.1 Headache prevalence as a function of age

Decrease in prevalence	Equally common	Increase in prevalence	Typically only in the elderly
Migraine	?Cluster headache	Intracranial lesions	Giant cell arteritis
Tension-type headache		Medication-induced (except rebound) headache	Hypnic headache
		'Metabolic headache' anaemia hypoxia hypercalcaemia hyponatraemia chronic renal failure	Headache of Parkinson's disease
		Cerebrovascular disease	

Modified from Edmeads and Takahashi, 1993.

Table 15.2 Common causes of headache beginning in late life

Secondary headache disorders	Primary headache disorders
Mass lesions	Migraine
Giant cell arteritis	Tension-type headache
Medication-related headaches	Cluster headache
Trigeminal neuralgia	Hypnic headache
Postherpetic neuralgia	
Systemic disease	
Disease of the cranium, neck, eyes, ears and nose	
Cerebrovascular disease	
Parkinson's disease	

elderly women; Figure 15.1). The most frequent metastatic tumours are lung and breast cancers, followed by malignant melanomas and carcinomas of the kidney and gastrointestinal tract. Pain patterns that result from primary and metastatic tumours vary. Headaches associated with brain tumours most often resemble TTH. The classic pattern of severe pain, early morning awakening, and nausea occurs in only 17% of patients with brain tumours. Headaches often develop before focal neurological signs and symptoms appear; thus neuroimaging is required in elderly patients with new-onset headaches.

Chronic SDH often act as mass lesions and may present with headache symptoms similar to those of a brain tumour. The elderly are at greater risk for SDH, in part caused by brain atrophy that decreases the support of bridging veins and causes tears and bleeding. Since SDH are extra-axial (outside the brain parenchyma), they are less likely to produce early neurological deficits. Some patients present with headache and confusion or a fluctuating level of consciousness. As SDH may present long after the trauma, a patient may deny a history of head injury, perhaps because it has been forgotten.

Giant cell arteritis

The systemic vasculitis GCA primarily affects medium-sized arteries. Signs and symptoms include headache, visual loss, fatigue, and myalgias. Rare before 50 years of age, the incidence of GCA increases dramatically after this, occurring in 3–9 per 100,000 population per year, with women affected three times more often than men.

The presence of GCA should be suspected in any elderly patient with new-onset headaches or a substantial change in headache pattern. Headache, the most frequent symptom, is present in 70–90% of GCA patients. The pain can be intermittent or constant and is often located over the temples. There is often associated scalp tenderness, especially over inflamed arteries. As a consequence, local pressure, such as wearing a hat or resting the head on a pillow, may exacerbate the pain (Table 15.3). Polymyalgia rheumatica, the symptoms of which include muscle pain and joint stiffness, is present in 25% of patients with GCA. Other common symptoms of GCA include fever, weight loss, night sweats, masseter claudication

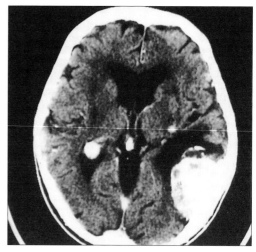

Figure 15.1 *Computed tomography of the brain illustrates meningioma arising in the left parietal region of an elderly woman. Since meningiomas arise from the dura mater, the tumours typically have a dural base as shown here.*

(pain with chewing), amaurosis fugax (may be bilateral in half of patients), permanent blindness (often without warning), or partial visual loss from anterior ischaemic optic neuropathy. Also, GCA should be included in the differential diagnosis of amaurosis fugax. Dysphoria, anorexia, and weight loss are common in GCA and may lead to a diagnosis of depression. Patients or physicians may mistakenly relate the onset of symptoms to a coincidental painful life event.

Visual loss is the most feared complication of GCA, occurring in about one-third of untreated patients. Visual loss is usually sudden and irreversible; however, gradual loss and recovery of vision with treatment have been reported. Visual

Table 15.3 *Symptoms and signs in giant cell arteritis*

Headache
Fatigue
Myalgia
Arthralgia
Depressed mood
Jaw claudication
Features of the temporal artery • tenderness • induration • diminished or absent pulse

loss is usually caused by ischaemic optic neuropathy secondary to arteritis of the blood vessels that supply the anterior optic nerve. In untreated cases, monocular visual loss may be followed by loss of vision in the other eye. Other ischaemic symptoms can occur. The pain of jaw claudication has a gradual onset compared with the rapid onset of the lancinating pain of trigeminal neuralgia. Ischaemia of the extraocular muscles and/or the oculomotor nerves may produce diplopia because of ocular motor paresis. Coronary, mesenteric, hepatic, and renal artery ischaemia have also been reported. Aortic arch syndrome may occur with rupture of the aorta. Stroke and transient ischaemic attack (TIA) can occur in GCA.

Induration and tenderness of the temporal or occipital scalp arteries are the most common signs of temporal arteritis. Visual fields and visual acuity should be assessed. Patients without visual loss have a normal funduscopic examination. In acute anterior ischaemic optic neuropathy, optic disc oedema and visual loss may occur. Arterial bruits or diminished pulses are present in one-third of patients.

The most consistent laboratory abnormality is an elevated Westergren ESR. The ESR may be reduced in patients who take aspirin, non-steroidal anti-inflammatory drugs (NSAIDs), or systemic corticosteroids, leading to a false-negative test. Elevated C-reactive protein, mild liver function abnormalities, and mild anaemia are also common.

Temporal artery biopsy is the diagnostic gold standard and should be performed within 48 hours of initiating corticosteroid treatment if possible. If the biopsy is negative (and this can occur because the disease can be patchy) and the index of suspicion remains high, additional sections from the first biopsy or a second, contralateral temporal artery biopsy may be diagnostic. Treatment should begin promptly while awaiting the results of the temporal artery biopsy in patients with a characteristic GCA profile and an elevated ESR (Figure 15.2).

The major goal of treatment is to prevent sudden, irreversible visual loss. Initial doses of prednisone range from 40 to 80 mg daily, and some experts employ intravenous corticosteroids for the first dose. Some investigators have suggested the use of megadose intravenous corticosteroids when unusual signs or symptoms are

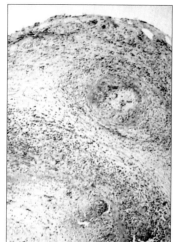

● **Figure 15.2**
Micrograph of a temporal artery biopsy in a patient with giant cell arteritis. (Reproduced with permission from Goadsby and Silberstein, 1997.)

present. The headache and the systemic symptoms typically remit shortly after treatment is started. After several weeks of therapy, the prednisone dose can be gradually reduced. A maintenance dose that controls symptoms should be maintained for 6 months to 1 year.

Medication-induced headache

Medications are an important cause of headache in the elderly (Table 15.4). Drugs may initiate a new type of headache or exacerbate a pre-existing headache disorder. Although a drug is associated with headache, it does not prove a causal role for a particular patient, and neither does it preclude the need to evaluate other causes. Medication withdrawal or rebound headaches may also occur.

● **Table 15.4** *Selected medications reported to cause headaches*

Amantadine	Monoamine oxidase inhibitors
Calcium-channel blockers	Non-steroidal anti-inflammatory agents
Caffeine	
Cimetidine	Nitrates
Corticosteroids	Nicotinic acid
Cyclophosphamide	Phenothiazines
Dipyridamole	Ranitidine
Oestrogens	Sympathomimetic agents
Ethanol	Tamoxifen
Hydralazine	Theophyllines (thioxanthines)
Indomethacin	Tetracyclines
L-Dopa	Trimethoprim

When medications trigger a pre-existing headache disorder, the headaches that are provoked are usually similar to the pre-existing headaches. Perhaps the most important pharmacological triggers of headache are alcohol and nitrate compounds, but antihypertensives are also common culprits in this age group. Nitroglycerin can induce both migraine and cluster attacks. Hormonal replacement therapy and food additives, such as monosodium glutamate, aspartate, caffeine, and tyramine, may increase headache frequency. Medication-withdrawal headaches (rebound headaches) are very common in headache subspecialty practices, although they may be less common in the elderly than in young adults.

Trigeminal neuralgia

Trigeminal neuralgia is the most common neuralgic syndrome in the elderly, with a peak incidence of 155 cases per million population and a female:male ratio of 3:2 (Table 15.5). It is typically unilateral, but is bilateral in 4% of patients. The pain is characterized by brief, unilateral paroxysms (similar to a spasm or electric shock) in one or more divisions of the trigeminal nerve. The pain may be provoked by stimulating specific trigger points or by stimuli, such as washing, shaving, talking, or brushing the teeth. The pain can precipitate facial paroxysms, which resulted in the condition being previously named *tic douloureux*, and may be followed by a sustained, deep, dull ache.

The aetiology of trigeminal neuralgia varies with age (Table 15.6). In the elderly, it is commonly thought to result from neurovascular compression of the trigeminal nerve caused by abnormal arterial loops near the trigeminal nerve root entry zone. Vascular compression leads to demyelination and aberrant neuronal activity, which may produce sensitization in the trigeminal nucleus caudalis.

The typical clinical features of trigeminal neuralgia establish the diagnosis. The physical examination is negative except for positive trigger points. Diagnostic studies are generally normal. Impaired sensation in the distribution of the Vth nerve suggests a structural, demyelinating, or compressive trigeminal nerve lesion (Table 15.6). The initial evaluation should include MRI, with special attention to the region of the cerebellopontine angle and the exit foramen of the trigeminal nerve.

If structural disease is absent, medical therapy should be initiated (Table 15.7). The initial drug of choice is carbamazepine, followed by valproate (divalproex), baclofen, and clonazepam. The newer compound, gabapentin, may also be helpful. If medication fails to adequately control the symptoms, ablative procedures should be considered, including alcohol or glycerol injections, gasserian ganglion or retrogasserian injec-

---

Table 15.5 *Idiopathic trigeminal neuralgia*

Diagnostic criteria

A Paroxysmal attacks of facial or frontal pain which last a few seconds to less than 2 minutes.

B Pain has at least four of the following characteristics:

  1 Distribution along one or more divisions of the trigeminal nerve.

  2 Sudden, intense, sharp, superficial, stabbing, or burning in quality.

  3 Pain intensity severe.

  4 Precipitation from trigger areas, or by certain daily activities such as eating, talking, washing the face, or cleaning the teeth.

  5 Between paroxysms the patient is entirely asymptomatic.

C No neurological deficit.

D Attacks are stereotyped in the individual patient.

E Exclusion of other causes of facial pain by history, physical examination, and special investigations.

From Headache Classification Committee of the International Headache Society, 1988.

Table 15.6 *Causes of trigeminal neuralgia*

A Decreased facial sensation

- Intracranial aneurysms
- Giant cell arteritis
- Intracranial tumours
- Dental mandibular malignancy
- Cranial malignancy

B Normal facial sensation

- Idiopathic trigeminal neuralgia (from vascular compression)
- Multiple sclerosis
- Dental pathology
- Dental procedures

Table 15.7 *Drug treatment of trigeminal neuralgia**

Drug	Bioavailability (%)	Time to maximum concentration (hrs)	Half-life (hrs)	Time to steady-state concentration (days)	Therapeutic 'target' range (mmol/l)
Baclofen	–	3–8	3–4	1	–
Carbamazepine	>70	2–8	11–27	5	24–43
Clonazepam	100	1–2	24–48	12	30–270
Lamotrigine	100	2–3	18–30	8	4–16
Oxcarbazepine	100	1–2	14–26	7	5–110
Phenytoin	98	4–8	15–20	14	20–80
Valproic acid	99	1–4	6–17	5	200–700

*Modified from Zakrzewski, 1995a, 1995b.

tions, radiofrequency or percutaneous bulbar gangliolysis, or microvascular decompression via occipital craniotomy. Recently, the gamma knife (focused beams of radiation) has been used to treat trigeminal neuralgia.

Glossopharyngeal neuralgia

Less common than trigeminal neuralgia, the unilateral pain of glossopharyngeal neuralgia occurs in the distribution of the glossopharyngeal and vagus nerves in and around the ear, jaw, throat, tongue, or larynx, commonly with radiation to the ear. Paroxysms of jabbing or electric pain may be followed by deep, continuous pain between paroxysms, and may number 30–40 attacks a day. Paroxysms of pain may be triggered by chewing, talking, yawning, coughing, swallowing cold liquids, or stimulating the auditory and postauricular areas. Syncope (secondary to bradycardia or asystole) and seizures (from cerebral ischaemia) can occur, but this is rare. The best diagnostic test is anaesthetization of the tonsil and pharynx, which can temporarily terminate a painful paroxysm and confirm the diagnosis. Pharmacotherapy is identical to the approach outlined for trigeminal neuralgia (Table 15.7). Surgical treatment involves intracranial sectioning of the glossopharyngeal nerve and the upper rootlets of the vagus nerve at the jugular foramen.

Postherpetic neuralgia

Postherpetic neuralgia (Table 15.8), a significant cause of head pain in the elderly, is defined by the presence of pain after the eruption of herpes zoster. Typical involvement in the head occurs unilaterally in the distribution of the ophthalmic or maxillary divisions of the trigeminal nerve, or at the occipitocervical junction. Ophthalmic herpes may be associated with diplopia from involvement of cranial nerves III, IV, and VI. Geniculate herpes is associated with facial palsy, and vesicles are often seen in the auditory canal. Many people have persistent pain after the herpes eruption clears. Age is a risk factor for postherpetic neuralgia, which occurs in 75% of those over 70 years of age, particularly when the acute attack of zoster is intense. Other risk factors include diabetes mellitus, an ophthalmic location for the eruption, and immunological compromise.

The pain of postherpetic neuralgia has three components:

- constant, deep burning pain;
- repetitive stabs and needle-pricking sensations; and
- superficial, sharp, or radiating pain or itching triggered by light touch.

The pain often remits, and after 3 years over half of the patients are free of troublesome pain. Topical therapies, such as Burow's solution compresses,

Table 15.8 *Chronic postherpetic neuralgia*

Diagnostic criteria

A Pain is restricted to the distribution of the affected cranial nerves or divisions thereof.

B Pain persists more than 6 months after the onset of herpetic eruption.

colloidal oatmeal, or calamine lotion, are used to treat acute zoster. Oral glucocorticoids may speed the resolution of acute zoster pain, but it is unclear whether they prevent postherpetic neuralgia. Antiviral agents may attenuate acute herpes zoster in immunocompromised patients. Although aciclovir has not been proved to reduce the risk of postherpetic neuralgia, a 21-day course of aciclovir may ameliorate pain in the acute phase. Famciclovir may shorten the duration of postherpetic neuralgia.

Postherpetic neuralgia should be treated as soon as the diagnosis is made. Amitriptyline is commonly used, but nortriptyline or desipramine may be preferable, since they have fewer anticholinergic side effects. Capsaicin, a topical agent that depletes substance P, is helpful, but the burning pain that sometimes accompanies its application may limit its usefulness. Topical NSAIDs may be useful, and local anaesthetic preparations have been used with some success. Peripheral and central surgical techniques are of little, if any, value.

Headaches associated with systemic disease

Headache can be a symptom of a systemic disease, some of which are more common in the elderly. Infection is the most common systemic cause. Although not age-related, viral and bacterial infections, as well as Lyme disease and other spirochete-caused diseases, can produce headache. Headache may be associated with acute Epstein–Barr virus and chronic fatigue syndrome. Other systemic diseases that cause headaches include acute (but not chronic) hypertension, hypercalcaemia, severe anaemia, and renal disease or its treatment (dialysis). Hypoxia or hypercapnia are more common in the elderly and may produce headache regardless of the cause, such as obstructive sleep apnoea. Pacemaker insertion or tumour involvement of the mediastinum may produce pain referred to the head through the autonomic nervous system.

Headache associated with disorders of the cranium, neck, eyes, ears, and nose

Primary disorders of the cranial bones are rare. Cervical spine abnormalities may produce anterior or posterior head pain, perhaps from involvement of the cervical nerve roots or descending trigeminal nerve tract. Typical clinical features of headache of cervical origin include:

- occipital or suboccipital pain, sometimes reproduced or augmented by suboccipital pressure;
- neck tenderness and muscle spasms that may produce limited movement, unusual postures, and pain with neck motion; and
- sensory abnormalities in the distribution of the upper cervical roots.

These headaches are usually unilateral. Many patients diagnosed with what has been called cervicogenic headache meet the criteria for migraine or TTH. It seems clear that, in addition to the many other trigger factors for migraine, cervical spine disease may be a particularly problematic one in the elderly.

Miotic eyedrops, such as pilocarpine, used to treat primary open-angle glaucoma may produce brow ache. Secondary angle-closure glaucoma resulting from diabetes or carotid insufficiency may produce a deep, boring, unrelenting eye pain with red eye and poor vision.

Inflammation or infection of the ear can produce headache. Middle or external ear infections can usually be diagnosed on routine examination. Acute sinusitis produces headache, usually with sinus tenderness, purulent nasal discharge, and perhaps fever. Infection of the teeth or mucous membranes of the mouth may cause pain in adjacent areas of the mouth or face, as well as head and facial pain.

Headaches associated with other neurological disorders

Cerebrovascular disease and Parkinson's disease may produce headache in the elderly. The headache of cerebrovascular disease may occur before, during, or after the onset of stroke or TIA. The headaches may occur with large vessel thrombotic stroke (20–40%), embolic stroke (20–40%), lacunar infarction (18%), subarachnoid haemorrhage (>95%), or intracerebral haemorrhage (80%). Headache may also follow carotid endarterectomy.

Parkinson's disease

The association between Parkinson's disease and headache is unclear, with one series reporting headache in 41% of Parkinson's disease patients and 13% of controls, and another series reporting no difference. Possible headache mechanisms include comorbid depression and muscle rigidity. In one study of early morning occipital headache in patients with Parkinson's disease, the headache failed to improve with treatment directed at muscle spasm, but it did improve with levodopa. These headaches may respond to amitriptyline.

Primary headache disorders in the elderly

Migraine headache

Although migraine prevalence peaks near 40 years of age, 5% of women and 2% of men over 70 years of age suffer from migraine. Only 2% of all migraine cases begin after 65 years of age; for this reason, caution is advised in diagnosing new-onset migraine in the elderly. Studies suggest that headache characteristics may change with advancing age. Migraine attacks may remit or evolve into chronic daily headache, with or without medication overuse. Migraine with aura may transform into a periodic neurological deficit with little or no headache pain, which is a phenomenon of aura without headache termed 'late-life migraine accompaniments'.

Features of late-life migraine accompaniments are listed in Table 15.9. Those most consistent with migraine are scintillations or other visual displays, slow (typically minutes) evolution of the neurological deficit, and serial progression from one symptom to another. Diagnosis is one of

exclusion. The neurological examination and neuroimaging studies are normal. Alternative diagnoses include cerebral thrombosis, embolism, TIA, carotid or vertebral dissection, subclavian steal syndrome, epilepsy, thrombocythaemia, polycythaemia, hyperviscosity syndrome, and lupus. Patients with late-life migraine accompaniments have normal angiograms and rarely develop permanent neurological deficits.

Medications that older patients commonly take can exacerbate pre-existing migraine or precipitate new migraine-like headaches. Common offenders include nitroglycerin compounds and oestrogen replacement therapy. Reducing the dose may ameliorate the headaches.

Acute migraine treatments should be used cautiously in elderly patients:

- ergot alkaloids and 5-hydroxytryptamine-1 agonists (triptans [sumatriptan, rizatriptan, electripan, naratriptan, and zolmitriptan]) may exacerbate pre-existing hypertension, coronary artery disease, peripheral vascular disease, or cerebrovascular disease, and may sometimes provoke ischaemic complications, including angina, myocardial infarction, or claudication;
- NSAIDs may cause peptic ulcer disease, gastrointestinal bleeding, or cognitive side effects in elderly patients and can potentially interact with anticoagulants, hypoglycaemics, digoxin, antihypertensive agents, and diuretics;
- antiemetic agents (such as metoclopramide and chlorpromazine) may cause extrapyramidal syndromes;
- benzodiazepines and barbiturates may cause excessive sedation – the long-acting benzodiazepines may cause excessive side effects from slowed metabolic clearance;
- tertiary amine tricyclic antidepressants (amitriptyline and doxepin), which are potent anticholinergic agents, may exacerbate glaucoma, produce visual blurring, and cause cognitive problems (instead use agents with minimal anticholinergic and sedative side effects, such as nortriptyline, which is a secondary amine with less fewer side effects);

● **Table 15.9** *Migraine equivalents*

- Gradual appearance of focal neurological symptoms – spread or intensification over a period of minutes.
- Positive visual symptoms characteristic of 'classic' migraine, specifically fortification spectra (scintillating scotoma), flashing lights, dazzles.
- Previous similar symptoms associated with a more severe headache.
- Serial progression from one accompaniment to another.
- The occurrence of two or more identical spells.
- A duration of 15–25 minutes.
- Occurrence of a 'flurry' of accompaniments.
- A generally benign course without permanent sequelae.

- selective serotonin reuptake inhibitors, although not as effective for migraine prophylaxis, are well tolerated by the elderly;
- antihypertensive drugs may cause more hypotension or lethargy;
- Methysergide and methylergonovine may cause cardiac ischaemia because they are vasoconstrictors, so they are relatively contraindicated; and
- sodium valproate has a particularly good benefit-to-side-effect profile.

The principles of migraine treatment outlined in Chapter 6 apply to the elderly; however, preventive treatments cause more side effects. The distribution and excretion of many medications are altered in the elderly patient, which generally results in higher blood levels for a given dose. The elderly are also more sensitive to anticholinergic, orthostatic, sedative, and cardiac side effects. Therefore, drugs should be started at a low dose and increased slowly.

Non-pharmacological treatment is attractive in the elderly patient, as it is in all patients, because it avoids medications that present risks or side effects. The following strategies are useful for all patients – eliminate triggers, maintain proper diet, maintain a regular sleep pattern, and avoid excess caffeine. Biofeedback may not be as effective in the elderly patient. It is very important to identify and treat comorbid medical and psychiatric conditions.

Tension-type headache

Tension-type headache (TTH) can begin at any age. It most commonly begins before 40 years of age, but in 10% of patients, it begins after 50. Medical disorders common in the elderly may be mistaken for TTH. The differential diagnosis includes mass lesions, temporal arteritis, visual acuity problems, and chronic daily headache that evolves from migraine.

Treatment of TTH should be modified in elderly patients. Combination analgesics contain sedatives or caffeine, and their use should be limited because overuse may cause dependence and more side effects. Preventive therapy should be administered when a patient has frequent headaches that produce disability or may lead to acute medication overuse. Antidepressants, which

are the type of medication of choice, should be started at a very low dose and increased slowly every 3–7 days. Selective serotonin reuptake inhibitors may be preferable to tricyclics.

Cluster headache

Although cluster headache typically begins between 20 and 50 years of age, onset of both the episodic and chronic varieties has been reported in patients in their eighties. Cluster attacks may persist or recur after many years of remission. Of the medications commonly used by the elderly, sublingual or transdermal nitroglycerin is a potent precipitator of cluster attacks.

Pharmacological treatment is influenced by the presence of comorbid medical conditions and the drugs used for treating them. When the patient does not have chronic obstructive pulmonary disease, oxygen inhalation may be the safest and most effective method of aborting attacks. The other mainstays to abort cluster headache – sumatriptan or ergotamine compounds – must be used very cautiously even in the absence of peripheral vascular disease, coronary heart disease, or hypertension.

We do not recommend methysergide for elderly patients. Verapamil, lithium, and prednisone should be used with caution. Sodium valproate is preferred.

Hypnic headaches

The hypnic headache syndrome is a rare primary headache disorder of the elderly with onset between 65 and 84 years of age and with no clear gender preponderance. Patients present with headaches that awaken them from sleep at the same time almost every night and last for 15–60 minutes. The pain is typically diffuse (but can be unilateral), often throbbing, and not associated with the autonomic features of cluster headaches. The headaches may be associated with rapid eye movement sleep (Table 15.10).

Hypnic headache must be differentiated from a mass lesion (which may also present with nocturnal pain) and from temporal arteritis. Cluster headaches also present with nocturnal attacks, but can be differentiated from hypnic headaches by their unilaterality, their periorbital and temporal location, and their prominent autonomic features.

After excluding organic disease with an imaging procedure and an ESR treatment with lithium carbonate, 300 mg at bedtime, usually produces a prompt remission of hypnic headache. If headaches recur, higher doses of lithium may be required, or verapamil given at bedtime (40–120 mg) can also be effective. Lithium should be used with caution in the elderly, especially in the presence of renal disease, dehydration, or diuretic therapy.

Table 15.10 *Suggested International Headache Society (IHS) diagnostic criteria for hypnic headache*

4.7 Hypnic headache

A Headaches occur at least 15 times per month for at least 1 month.

B Headaches awaken patient from sleep.

C Attack duration of 5–60 minutes.

D Pain is generalized or bilateral.

E Pain is not associated with autonomic features.

F At least one of the following:

- There is no suggestion of one of the disorders listed in IHS groups 5–11.
- Such a disorder is suggested but excluded by appropriate investigations.
- Such a disorder is present, but the first headache attacks do not occur in close temporal relation to the disorder.

Modified from Goadsby and Lipton, 1997.

Summary

- The physician must search for an underlying cause when an elderly patient presents with a new-onset headache. If a cause is identified, treatment should consider both the underlying cause and the pain syndrome. For the patient in whom secondary headaches are excluded, a specific primary headache disorder should be diagnosed.
- Treatment goals include pain prevention, pain relief, and optimal functioning and quality of life.
- Pharmaceutical treatment must be selected cautiously, taking into consideration any comorbid conditions and possible drug interactions.

Further reading

Edmeads J, Takahashi A. Headache in the elderly. In: Olesen J, Tfelt-Hansen P, Welch KMA (eds). *The Headaches.* New York: Raven Press, 1993: 809–13.

Forsyth PA, Posner JB. Headaches in patients with brain tumors. A study of 111 patients. *Neurology* 1993; 43: 1678– 83.

Fisher CM. Late-life migraine accompaniments as a cause of unexplained transient ischemia attacks. *Can J Neurol Sci* 1980; 7 :9–17.

Goadsby PJ, Lipton RB. A review of paroxysmal hemicranias, SUNCT syndrome and other short lasting headaches with autonomic features, including new cases. *Brain* 1997: 120; 193–209.

Goadsby PJ, Silberstein SD (eds). *Headache.* Boston: Butterworth–Heinemann, 1997.

Headache Classification Committee of the International Headache Society. Classification and diagnostic criteria for headache disorders, cranial neuralgia, and facial pain. *Cephalalgia* 1988; 8(7): 19–6.

Kost RG, Straus SE. Postherpetic neuralgia – pathogenesis, treatment, and prevention. *N Engl J Med* 1996; 335: 32–42.

Lipton RB, Pfeffer D, Newman L, Solomon S. Headaches in the elderly. *J Pain Symptom Manage* 1993; 8: 87–97.

Silberstein SD, Young WB. Headache. In: Pathy MSJ (ed). *Principles and Practices of Geriatric Medicine,* 3rd edn. New York: John Wiley & Sons, 1998: 733–46.

Swannell AJ. Fortnightly review: polymyalgia rheumatica and temporal arteritis: diagnosis and management. *BMJ* 1997: 314, 1329–32.

Zakrzewska JM. Perpheral surgery. In: Trigeminal neuralgia. *Major Problems in Neurology.* London: WB Saunders, 1995a: 108–55.

Zakrzewska JM. Posterior fossa surgery. In: Trigeminal neuralgia. *Major Problems in Neurology.* London: WB Saunders, 1995b: 157–70.

Index